JN184886

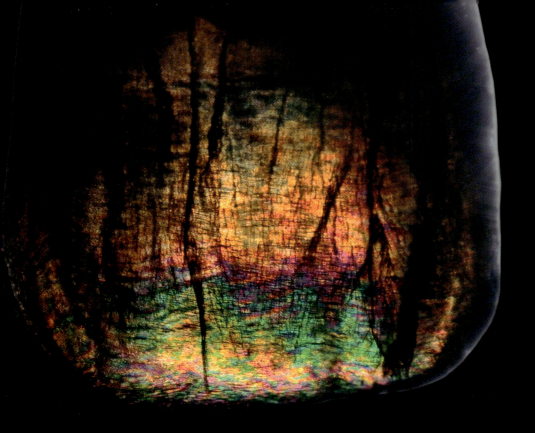

Color and internal shape of Anteriores

Impact

山本尚吾 著

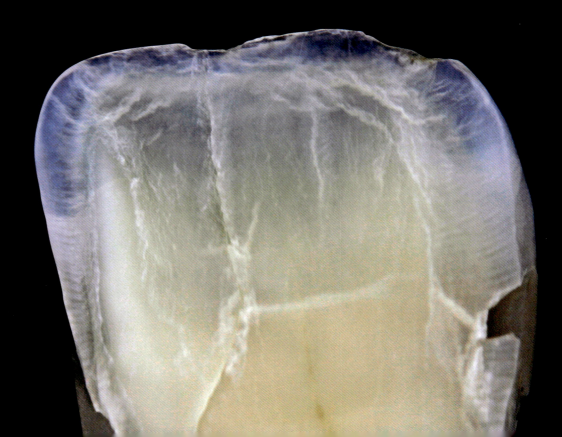

医歯薬出版株式会社
http://www.ishiyaku.co.jp/

This book was originally published in Japanese
under the title of :

IMPAKUTO KARA ANDO INTANARU SHIEIPU OBU ANTERIASU
Impact Color and internal shape of Anteriores

Author :

SHOGO, Yamamoto

© 2017   1st ed.

ISHIYAKU PUBLISHERS, INC.
  7-10 Honkomagome 1 chome, Bunkyo-ku,
  Tokyo 113-8612, Japan

序文

　本書は，筆者にとって初めて著す単行本である．そして，筆者が歯科技工に従事した30年の間に収集した，日本人の上顎前歯部の抜去天然歯をそのままの姿で，または唇舌的に割断したり，エナメル質のみを削除したり，象牙質のみを削除したりして，それらを光学的及び構造的に観察した写真集である．

　補綴治療において，特に色調が天然歯に近似した補綴物を製作するという目的のために，ターゲットとなる天然歯の象牙質の構造及びエナメル質の光学的な"秘密"を知りたいと思うのは，筆者だけではないと思う．筆者もその思いを絶やすことなく，可能な限りサンプルとなる天然歯を収集してきた．このサンプルの天然歯を集めることが，前述の秘密を知るうえで最大の重要事であることは，読者諸氏にはご理解いただけるであろう．筆者が過去に勤務した歯科医院で抜去歯を譲ってもらったり，歯科技工所開業後には取引先の歯科医院に無理を言って集めてもらったり，友人である歯科医師にプレゼントされたり……．筆者はサンプルを収集することにおいて，とてもラッキーだったように思う．今さらではあるが，筆者のサンプルの収集に尽力してくださった友人諸氏及び歯科医師の先生がたに，この場を借りて改めて御礼を述べたい．

　また，せっかく収集した天然歯を被写体として，可能な限り良い仕上がりが得られるように撮影を心掛けたのだが，カメラの技術的な事由において思い通りの撮影ができなかったり，天然歯を切削する等の操作中に壊してしまったりする等，作業は決して容易いものではなかった．いずれにせよ，様々な観点から観察や考察ができるような写真集とすることを企図したが，撮影が進むにつれて，筆者が過去に撮影を終えて満足していた天然歯のサンプルについても再度撮影に挑戦したいと思うようになり，観察と撮影に没頭しては，膨大な画像データの中から良い仕上がりの写真を選ぶことに疲れ果てる日々でもあった（その労苦は今でも鮮明に思い出される）．それでも，過去に撮影したサンプルを今改めて撮影し直してみると，新たな発見も得られた．なるべく主観にとらわれないように気を付けて撮影作業を進めたが，あくまで狭い世界での記録であるため，筆者の主観が多く含まれることも否めないのではあるが，筆者なりに天然歯を観察し，特に本書では歯に入射した光の透過と拡散及び，象牙質の構造等を捉えることを主眼に置いた．中でも，筆者がこれまで"理屈"のみで解釈していた象牙質とエナメル質の見事なまでのコラボレーションを撮影し表現できたことで，筆者自身のセラミックス技工における表現法にまつわる多くのアイデアとヒントを得られた．まさにインスピレーションを得る瞬間を多く経験できたのである．

　材質及び光学特性においても相反する象牙質とエナメル質との調和により織り成される歯の色調も，光がなければ発色することはできない．まさに月と同じで，自らが光り輝くことはできないのだ．臨床の傍ら，天然歯のサンプル撮影に明け暮れる日々の中，ふと見上げた夜空に奇麗な月が輝いていた．さっそく超望遠撮影ができるカメラを三脚に固定して月の満ち欠けや時間ごとの変化を撮影する日が始まってしまった．しかしそのおかげで，自然からもセラミックスワークにおける大きなヒントを得ることができた．私感ではあるが，時折ページに掲載した月の写真には，特に光の反射と象牙質の性状との関連性を持たせてある．それらも合わせて楽しんでいただければ幸いである．

　本書を見ることによって，より多くの臨床家の方がたにインスピレーションを感じていただき，ダイレクトボンディングを行う歯科医師やセラミックス技工に従事する歯科技工士の読者諸氏にとって何らかのヒントとインパクトを与えられたならば心より嬉しく思う．

2017年　東京
山本尚吾

Preface

This is the first special photo book for me. This photo collection is mainly focusing on the observation of Japanese upper anterior teeth collected from over 30 years. The observation was done under refract and translucent light, cross sectional view of buccolingually, and only enamel or dentin part from the view point of structurally and optically. To create prosthesis as natural teeth, ceramist want to understand the optical secret of the tooth, as I want. The extracted natural anterior teeth have been collecting order of my desire of knowledge. The first important step, to collect the extracted anterior teeth without any caries and/or defects is the toughest work as you understand easily. I was very lucky for collecting them, because many dentists who have been working with me bring them. Such a wonderful situation, I would like to say thank to all of my friends.

The second big challenge is to show beautiful teeth truly in the printed book. My photo technique was not enough to visualize natural teeth same as my images on the picture, and digital camera required me to be higher level. In accordance with increase of my photo skill, new desire was come to me. I wanted to upgrade older pictures. After rebuild my photo collections, a lot of new findings were observed. In my mind, it might be better for readers to show many different faces. But sometime, I upset to select valuable one form huge amount of pictures. This is also good memory for me. The other technical problems were happened while in the removing process of enamel or dentin. Some valuable teeth were broken, it was very sad story. It was fun, but not very easy. The art of natural teeth in the tiny space, the nature of teeth should be shown as an objective analysis. Thus in this book, I really forces on objective point of view. I'm not sure that all readers enjoy it, but I hope you will find new image of natural structure of teeth under transmitted and reflect light.

In this book, the art of natural teeth was pointed out. Those understanding was constructed very logically. However, just a simple and careful observation of the micro photo gives me new ideas of ceramic work. It was easy to understand the relationship of dentin and enamel which from different light properties. The tooth structure never has shown the beautiful color without the light, like a moon. While in the clinical work, I took huge amount of pictures, and then suddenly I saw the lovely moon in the dark sky. I had started to take a different face of the moon naturally. I felt it was destiny. The moon also gives new images. Sometime, you can find the picture of different face of moon, it gives also you to find new imagination. I hope that the book will gives some new inspirations and impacts to all dentists and ceramists who work with art of fabulous aesthetic.

2017 Tokyo
Shogo Yamamoto

序

本書是筆者首次出版的牙科專業書籍，刊載了三十年來所匯集的日本人上顎前齒，皆是拔牙後的天然牙再進行加工切割去除琺瑯質、象牙質，以方便觀察天然牙的光學原理及構造本身．

為了使製作的補綴物可以接近所觀察的天然牙，對於牙體本身的琺瑯質光學原理以及象牙質構造，相信讀者們也跟筆者一樣感到好奇．

因此，首要工作就是盡可能的收集這些天然牙，好好保存做為參考樣本，希望讀者了解到這個重要性．我們可以向過去所服務過的醫療院所，或是開業後的客戶，乃至向牙醫師友人要求這樣的禮物，可以得到這些樣本對於筆者而言是非常幸運的．所以，在這裡也特別再次地向這些幫忙收集到樣本的朋友以及醫師們表達感謝之意．

緊接著的工作，即是費盡心思地想將寶貴的天然牙拍攝下來．不過，也許會受限於攝影技術，亦或是天然牙在切削過程中導致損壞，過程中不那麼盡如人意．不過，過去也有拍攝方式一改變之後，就有了新發現的經驗．另外，有時思考著要拍一些可以從不同面相來進行觀察或考察的照片，可是在拍攝的當下，又想再次挑戰一下先前認為拍得不錯的照片，一味地沉浸於觀察和拍攝，結果就會需要在大量圖庫中進行挑選，諸如此類回憶依然烙印腦中．當然需要小心翼翼地盡可能不被主觀想法影響，沉浸在這個狹小世界裡，無可厚非會有筆者主觀意識，因此本書也許有些無法滿足到讀者的地方．這次特別是光的穿透性和擴散性以及象牙質的構造等，將這些筆者所觀察到的予以刊載．

本書聚焦在天然牙的色調方面，以攝影呈現理論上象牙質與琺瑯質的相互關係，同時想著如何進行陶材表現，這樣的畫面會浮現在筆者的腦海，像是瞬間吸取到了許多創作靈感一般．

把材料及光學特性相反的象牙質，琺瑯質調和後，其實如果沒有光，所交織出的色調也就不可能呈現，亦如同天上的月娘也無法自己散發出光亮．某一天，一如往常地拍攝著樣本，不經意望上皎潔的明月，當下，使我馬上準備起腳架，架起了超望遠的鏡頭，這天我開始記錄起天上月的圓與缺．隨著這樣的一個契機，讓我又從大自然當中得到了陶瓷工作上的啟示．本書裡刊載了月的照片，可以體會一下特別是光的反射或是象牙質本身的表面性狀，均伴隨著某些意義，希望整合這些與讀者們分享．

無論是進行 Direct Bonding 的醫師，或是使用 ceramics 再現色調的牙技師們，希望帶給翻閱本書的臨床各位一些靈感與啟發，這將是我的榮幸．

2017年 東京
山本尚吾

Impact
Color and internal shape of Anteriores

Contents

序文 ··· 3

推薦文 ·· 8

Part 1
Maxillary central incisor and Lateral incisor ············· 16

Part 2-1
Internal structure and optical properties of maxillary anterior teeth · 22

Part 2-2
Fluorescence ··· 30

Part 3
Prologue **Linked to Palatal** ································· 38
  -The influence of tooth crown colors according to
  3 types of internal structure

Part 3-1
Mamelon Type ·· 46

Part 3-2
Mamelon Type + Box Type ···································· 56

Part 3-3
Box Type ·· 58

Part 3-4
Alteration ··· 66

Part 3-5
Anterior Root ··· 76

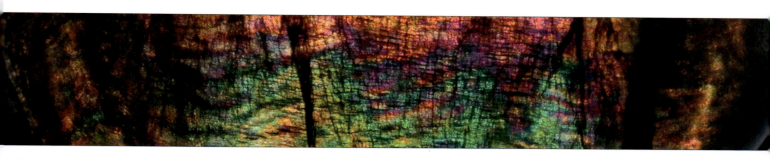

Part 4-1
Devil Head M Type ··· 86

Part 4-2
Devil Head B Type ··· 92

Part 5
Taper Type ··· 98

Part 6
Enamel ··· 104

Part 7
Lateral incisor ··· 124

Part 8
Canine ·· 126

Part 9
Lower anteriores ·· 134

Appendix ·· 138

Special Thanks ·· 142

Designed by a-pex design (Yasunori Sato)

推薦文 Testimonial

　私が初めて山本尚吾氏（show）と出会ったのは，1989年に京都で開催された，QZ社の主催する国際歯科技工学会においてであった．私にとっての彼の第一印象は，才能に満ち溢れ，何より天然歯における"光の行方"を熱心に追い求める努力家，であった．その出会い以来，彼は私が開催するセラミックスコースやフォトコースを何度も受講してくれ，そして私を何度も日本に招待し，素晴らしい景色を見せてくれたのだった．
　彼は，私が主催するグループ「art&experience®」の大切なメンバーである．彼のとどまるところを知らない研究心と探究心が，その名を世界中に知らしめるに至っていることについては，多言を要しないであろう．
　自然感を有する審美補綴装置の製作工程の多くが新しいデジタル技術に置き換わろうとするこの時代にこそ，彼が

　I first met Show Yamamoto at the QZ convention International Dental Technology Meeting 1989 in Kyoto, Japan. My first impressions of Show was that he seemed like a talented and eager dental technician who was striving to discover the behavior of light in the natural tooth structure. Since then he has attended many of my ceramic and photo courses and has invited me numerous times to Japan.
　Show has become a valuable art&experience® member. He has never lost his thirst for research and exploration in the dental world and due to that he has gained recognition globally.
　This book "INSPIRATION" from Show Yamamoto is notably valuable during this new digital age for

　我在1989年日本京都國際牙科技術會議QZ大會上第一次遇到Show Yamamoto．我對Show的第一印象是他看來是個致力於找出天然牙結構裡光的行為，深具才能和態度積極的牙科技師．從那時起他就參加許多我的陶瓷和照片課程，並邀請我去日本無數次．
　Show 已是 Art & Experience ® 裡具有價值的會員．他從來沒有失去對牙醫界的研究和探索渴望，也因此獲得全球認可．
　這本Show Yamamoto寫的書"INSPIRATION"在這個新數位時代，對那些想創造自然美學的人特別有價值．我很

著した本書にはとりわけ価値がある．私は，彼と出会い，過ごした時間から多くの着想を得られたことに心よりの感謝と敬意を表する．そして，傑出した歯科技工士であり，何より私の大切な友人である彼のためにこの推薦文を寄せる栄誉に浴することができたことを，とても誇りに思う．

スイス・バーゼル
Atelier Claude Sieber
Claude Sieber

all those who want to create natural aesthetics. I am honored that I was able to be an inspiration for him throughout all these years and I am proud to have had the privilege to write this foreword for Show Yamamoto, an outstanding technician and dear friend.

Basel, Switzerland
Atelier Claude Sieber
Claude Sieber

榮幸這些年能成為他的靈感來源，也很自豪擁有特權為Show Yamamoto，一個傑出的技術人員和親愛的朋友書寫本書的前言．

瑞士・巴塞爾
Atelier Claude Sieber
Claude Sieber

推薦文　Testimonial

　未だかつて見られない，天然歯の観察を様々な角度から行い，分析した名著が上梓された．まさにタイトルにふさわしい"Impact"を我々歯科医師及び歯科技工士に与える内容である．過去において確かに天然歯を観察し，集計した本はいくつか散見されるが，果たしてこれほどまでに細部にわたり分析したものがかつて存在したであろうか．

　これだけの数の天然歯（前歯）を収集するだけでも並大抵のことではないのに，形式・分類ごとに分けてそれぞれ集積するには，長い年月と地道な努力がなければ成されるものではない．

　特に印象的であったのは，著者が序文において，歯の観察に疲れてふっと空を見上げたところ，「夜空に月が見え，その美しさに感動し，それが天然歯の構造・色調（光の反射と象牙質の性状）と似通っていると認識した」と述べていたことである．

　本書は上顎中切歯を中心に内部構造と光の透過性，フロールエッセンス（蛍光性）から始まり，天然歯のストラクチャー（内部構造）を3つに分類し，それぞれについて解説している．

　A notable book was published, which was ever not seen, and in which natural teeth are observed and analyzed in wide angle. It has the contents which can give us, dentists and dental technicians "Impact" suitable for the title of this book. We can certainly find some books in the past, which have observed and summarized natural teeth, however we do not know whether there were such a book analyzed natural teeth so deep in detail.

　It is really hard work to collect natural teeth (front teeth) in such quantity, and moreover this great achievement of integrating the record divided into each type and classification could not be realized without any persistent effort for many years.

　What especially impressive was that the author said in the preface, looking up the sky in his fatigue of observing so many teeth, he said, "Looking up the moon in the night sky and being impressed with the beauty, I could perceive that it is very similar to the construction and color tone of natural tooth (the reflection of light and the character of Dentin)."

　Starting from the internal construction and the transparency of light taking the focus on Maxillary Upper Central Incisor and Fluorescence, this book classifies the structure of natural tooth into 3 parts

　本著作以前所未見天然牙的各種角度觀察與分析，呼應標題"Impact"予以呈現給牙醫師與牙技師．過去雖有類似觀察天然牙的相關書籍，然而本著作於細部分析上應實屬空前．

　作者得以收集到相當數量的天然牙前牙並非是件容易的事，匯整之後再進行各別分類，確實是一步步長年累月踏實努力所得到的結果．特別印象深刻的是序文中所提到，作者在觀察牙齒的疲憊之餘俯瞰著天空，深深地受到皎潔明月之美所感動，也因此聯想到天然牙構造和色調（光反射以及象牙質性狀），其大自然的相似性．

　本書從上顎中門齒開始，從內部構造和透光性以及螢光性等，以此三種分類進行分析解說，特別在Part3-5精闢分析了牙根階段性切片，說明牙髓的型態以及光的穿透範圍．也緊接著進行側門齒和犬齒，以及下顎前齒的解說與分析．

出色なのは，Part3-5において示されているように，歯根を各段階にスライスし，歯髄の形態及び光の透過限界を調べたことにある．その後も，側切歯，犬歯及び下顎前歯について，次々と観察・解説・解読を試みている．

　いずれにしても，本書は写真のクオリティも非常に高く，歯科医療従事者としては「見ているだけ」で楽しくなる．読み方，見方は個々の読者に，自由に委ねられている．そして本書を見れば，審美回復治療の難しさをも良く知ることになるだろう．

東京都渋谷区
原宿デンタルオフィス
山﨑長郎

and explains those respectively in detail.

It can be regarded as outstanding that, as indicated Part 3-5, tooth root was sliced into each phase, and the structure of Dental Pulp and the transparency limit of light were investigated.

In addition to this, focusing on Lateral Incisor, Canine and Mandibular Front Tooth, all the detail was observed, explained and deciphered.

In any case, this book has the high quality of the pictures and will make all the member engaged in dental works pleasant only by looking at the pictures. It is freely left to the readers how to read and understand this book, and all the reader would come to undersand through this book how delicate the esthetic recovery treatment is.

Shibuya-ku, Tokyo
HARAJUKU DENTAL OFFICE
Masao Yamazaki

　整體上本書以高品質的圖像方式呈現，對於牙科從業人員來說，無非是一道道的視覺饗宴．同時各位讀者享受之餘，多少也能體會一下美學治療時的困難度．

東京都渋谷区
原宿牙科诊所
山﨑長郎

推薦文 Testimonial

　山本尚吾氏について語るということ，それはすなわち，彼の歯科技工士としての営みを通じて撮影された卓越なる芸術写真の世界に我々を導いてしまうという，彼の才能を探し求めるという試みなのだ．芸術分野においてもそうであるように，彼が撮影したイメージには，視覚的な直感によって人びとを魅了する力があり，それは彼が製作するセラミックス修復物によって素晴らしい審美性が回復されることにもつながっている．

　そして我々は彼の中に，ある天賦の才を見出すことができる．それは，歯科医師と患者がそれぞれの立場にあって抱いている補綴治療に対する要望と期待を聞き届け，理解し，歯科矯正臨床に熟達した術者を交えたアプローチによって，補綴治療を成功に導くというものだ．

　彼は"自然"を模倣し，完璧な品位と美を備えた写真としてそれを我々に示してくれる．そして，「審美的成果における機能を捉えること」を主目的に掲げて彼が歯科技工士として歩む"道"は，形態，構造，表面性状，セラミックス材料の厚みといった諸要素を分析することによって"具現化"される．事実，審美的成果とは前述したそれぞ

　Speaking of Show Yamamoto means investigating a talent which takes us, through incredible photographic art, to the excellence of his works.

　For of art we are speaking, in both cases, where the ability is in capturing a visual intuition from an image, and restoring the great beauty of a ceramic artifact.

　In him we can observe this gift of listening and translating a vision which originates between doctor and patient, between desire and expectations which encounter each other and find, in the mastery of an orthodontic, the link which unites them.

　Yamamoto manages to imitate nature and give us shots which describe perfection, a state of grace and beauty.

　His path is realized through an accurate analysis of form, weaving, surfaces and the thickness of ceramic materials to capture the function in the aesthetic result, the primary objective in our itinerary.

　說到Show Yamamoto，意味透過令人難以置信的攝影藝術帶領我們接近他卓越作品的一個人才．對於我們所說的藝術，有從影像捕獲視直覺，並修復極美陶瓷製品的能力等兩種情況．

　在他身上，我們可以觀察到這種傾聽及轉換源於醫生和病人之間，彼此面對想望和期待之願景的天賦，並在精通齒列矯正中找到兩者之間的連結．

　Yamamoto模仿自然，給我們帶來描述完美—優雅和美麗狀態的照片．

　他透過對形狀，穿行，表面和陶瓷材料厚度的精確分析來實現他的方法，以捕獲美學結果的功能，這也是我們研究過程的主要目的。

　事實上，美學結果只能透過對每個單一元素本身具有的功能做出正確研究來實現．

れの要素が持つ機能に関する正しい研究・考究によってこそ達成できるのだ．そして彼は，自身が撮影した，歯肉における毛細血管まで鮮明に見えるようなミクロの世界を捉えた写真からの分析によって，審美と機能のバランスを兼ね備えた形態を有する"本物の彫像"としての補綴装置を作り出している．

彼の持つ好奇心に満ちた目とすべてを知り尽くした手……，そこから撮影された写真によって構成される本書は，最新の歯科技術を用いながらも，我々の従事する歯科医療において機械ではなく人間が関わることでより可能性が広がることを知る者，患者の幸福に対する献身と考究を続けるすべての者にとっての教導書となるであろう．

イタリア・ミラノ
Studio medico Gandini e Massironi
Domenico Massironi

In fact, the aesthetic result can only be achieved by the correct study of the function that each single element has in itself.

Through a capillary analysis, Yamamoto creates real 'sculptures' in which the aesthetic/functional balance takes form.

This books teaches, through curious eyes and knowing hands; to all those who still have the wish to nuture that human factor in our work, which uses modern technology, but remains anchored in a dimension of research, commitment and dedication to the wellbeing of the patient.

Milano, Italy
Studio medico Gandini e Massironi
Domenico Massironi

通過毛細管分析，Yamamoto創造了真正的"雕塑"，其中具有美學/功能平衡形式．

這本書透過好奇的眼睛和靈巧雙手，教導所有那些仍然希望在我們的工作中使用現代技術呈現自然的人類因素，但仍然堅持研究病人的福祉，並對之承諾和奉獻的人．

米蘭・義大利
Studio medico Gandini e Massironi
Domenico Massironi

推薦文 Testimonial

　私が山本尚吾（Show）氏との知遇を得たのは，台湾の歯科商社であるTESCO社とのあるミーティングにおいてであった．そして，初めて氏の講習会を受講した時，その独特なスタイルを深く実感し，さらに新たなデジタルテクニックによる歯科芸術を展開していることを認識した．氏の素晴らしい技術を勉強するために，私は当院の院内歯科技工士と歯科医師を集めて，東京にある氏のアトリエでその技術を学ぶセミナー開催を依頼し，デジタルテクニックを応用した前歯のセラミックス補綴装置の製作法を学んだ．そこから始まった私と氏との関係により，実際の患者の治療を行う臨床例を依頼し，実践での製作法を学びながら，術前の前準備，シェードテイキング，マテリアル（材料）の選択，デジタルデザイン等，これまでのデジタルテクニックの応用とは異なった観点からの製作法により具現化されたセラミックスクラウン補綴装置を見ることができた．私と山本氏で取り組んだ最初のケースには驚きを隠せなかった．なぜなら，私の目の前にはこれまで見たことない芸術作品があったのだ……．そして，目で見える芸術以外の，目に見えない細かなもの（歯の個性表現）も氏の手によって表現されており，これこそが歯科用CAD/CAMシステムを応用した審美補綴成功への鍵だと実感した．

　今日まで，歯科用CAD/CAMシステムをチェアサイドのみで応用する歯科医師は，"それなり"のセラミックスクラウンを製作することはできても，審美的なセラミックスクラウンを製作することは難しいと感じていた．しかし，山本氏と知り合うことができてからは，歯科技工士との協働によるセラミックスクラウン製作の基礎と術前の前準備

　When I first met Show sensei at one of his lectures, his stylistic and fiery passion left a deep and memorable impression. Immediately afterward, I reached out to be introduced to this wonderful instructor, and thus opened a door to a whole new world of dental arts. It quickly became apparent that his teachings would be tremendously helpful to others as well, and so I sent my own dental technicians to Japan as apprentices to study from the Show sensei. Happily, this would mark the beginning of our numerous and subsequent cooperative efforts.

　Even with extensive clinical experience, I am consistently amazed by the quality and artistic nature of our collaborated cases. Show Sensei's works have shown me that underneath every piece of art, its success lies in the attention to the finest details. At the same time, he demonstrates that truly functional and aesthetic dentures are indeed possible with CAD/CAM, contrary to popular belief. In

　認識 Show 老師是在一次與豐達牙材聊天的時候提到的，那個時候第一次參與 Show 老師的課程，就深深的被那種強烈又獨具風格的方式所吸引，那個時候就與豐達牙材接洽，希望能透過他們認識 Show 老師，認識 Show 老師之後，真正認知道全新的牙科藝術．

　為了學習 Show 老師的精湛技術，我們特地把診所的技師與醫師送到日本去跟老師拜師學習，也開啟了我們多次的合作機會．第一次與 Show 老師合作 Case 的時候真的是令我們非常的震驚，因為我們雖然曾經看過無數的 Case，但是從沒有機會看到這樣的藝術擺在眼前，也真正的體驗到，每一個完美，背後的細節，是真正成功的關鍵．

　曾經有很多醫師都覺得 CAD/CAM 無法真正的做出好的牙齒，但是直到認識 Show 老師之後，我們知道，這一切都是可能，而且 Show 老師在搭配使用 CAD/CAM 之後，能夠讓傳統的牙技師的技藝，更好呈現在牙科的美學之中得到

の重要性を改めて感じると共に,最新の歯科用CAD/CAMシステムを用いることと,歯科技工士の技術を融合させることにより,究極の審美歯科の再現が可能となることを実感した.山本氏は真面目に患者の声に真摯に耳を傾け,そして例え言語(日本語と台湾語)による意思疎通の不自由があろうと,非常に辛抱強くコミュニケーションを行い,写真を撮影し,シェードテイキングを行い,細かい形態の再現に集中した.山本氏は私に次のような言葉を教えてくれた.「私は自分の愛する人として患者に接し,美しさや微笑み,及び機能への考察に焦点を合わせます.患者のhappinessはすなわち我々のhappinessなのですから」.クラウンを装着した患者が鏡の中にいる自身を目にした瞬間,すべての答えがそこに現れていた.

このたび,山本氏が学び続けている天然歯を長期にわたり収集し,細かく撮影し,一冊の本として完成したことは,我々歯科医療従事者に多くのヒントを与えてくれるだろう.本書の完成を心から喜び,多くの歯科医師,歯科技工士にも目にしてほしいと思う.

台湾台北
Sweet Space Dental Clinic 院長,Cerec Asia 創立者
曹 皓崴

fact, his digital work flow serves as the complimentary canvas on which traditional skills from dental technicians can truly shine.

Show Sensei is a patient and disciplined practitioner, and despite language barrier, he endeavors to fully collect every piece of necessary clinical detail to create a masterpiece. Whenever I see the lucid satisfaction of our patients after delivering his work of art, I am reminded of the something he had once said.

"Imagine the patients to be our lovers. Focus on their beauty and their smile," he had told me. "Only when our lovers are happy, can we be happy, too."

Taipei, Taiwan
曹 皓崴

完美的詮釋.

在合作之中,我們看到Show老師十分認真的與病患溝通並且傾聽患者的聲音,就算有語言上的困難,Show老師也拿出十足的耐心與細節,專注每個拍照,比色,形態的細節.

Show老師說:『要把病患當成自己的愛人,專注於她的美,她的微笑,只有當病患開心,我們才會真正的快樂.』當牙齒完成後,放在病患的口中,病患看到鏡子的那一個瞬間,我想老師的一切堅持,都得到了答案.

Show老師,傳統與數位牙科結合的完美演繹.
台灣台北 悅庭診所院長暨Cerec Asia創辦人　曹皓崴醫師

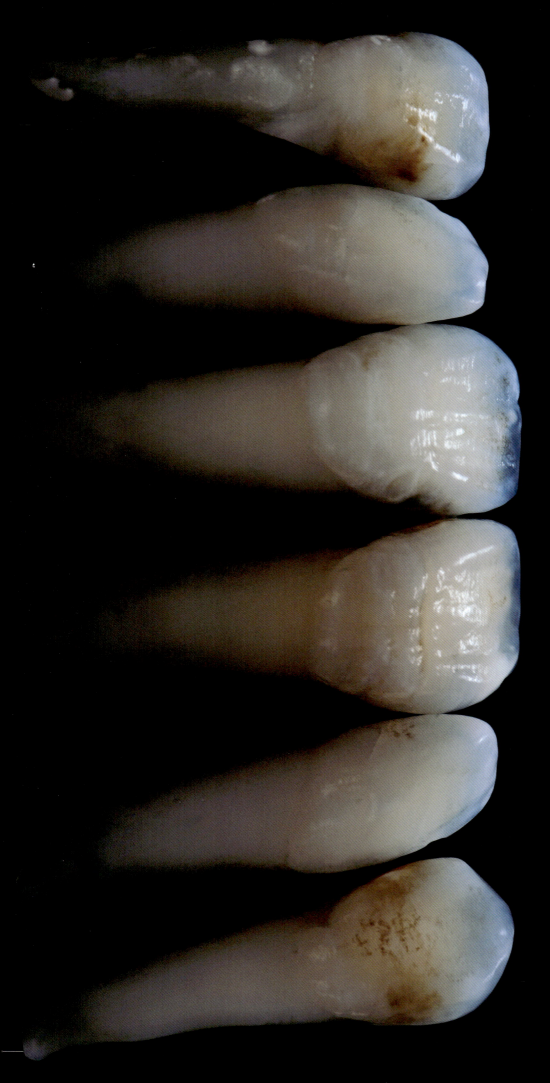

Part 1 Maxillary central incisor and

上顎前歯部が見せる表情．ラッキーなことに，筆者は同一患者の前歯部をサンプルとして収集することができた．

The harmony of maxillary anterior teeth. Luckily, I got six pears of maxillary incisors from single patients.

上顎前齒部的呈現．幸運地完成了患者前齒部位的樣本．

Lateral incisor

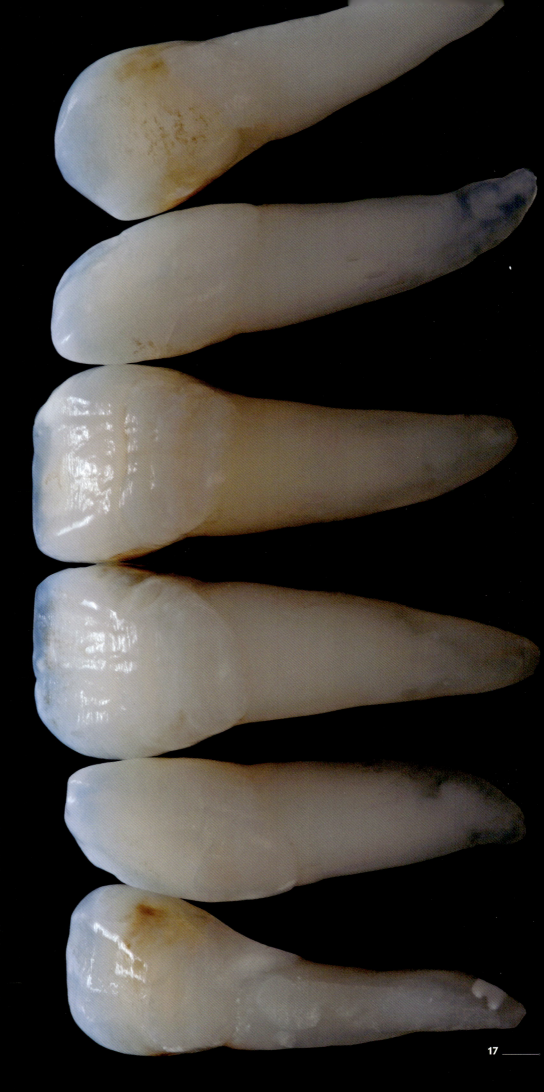

上顎前歯部は光の影響を受けやすい部位にある．光を受けることで白く輝く前歯部の再現は，セラミストにとっては永遠のテーマであろう．

Maxillary anterior region is the most affected part under the light influence. Blight lights natural teeth is the main dream for the dental ceramists.

上顎前歯部易受到光的影響，光線中所呈現出晶瑩潔白的前牙，這是Ceramist的永遠課題．

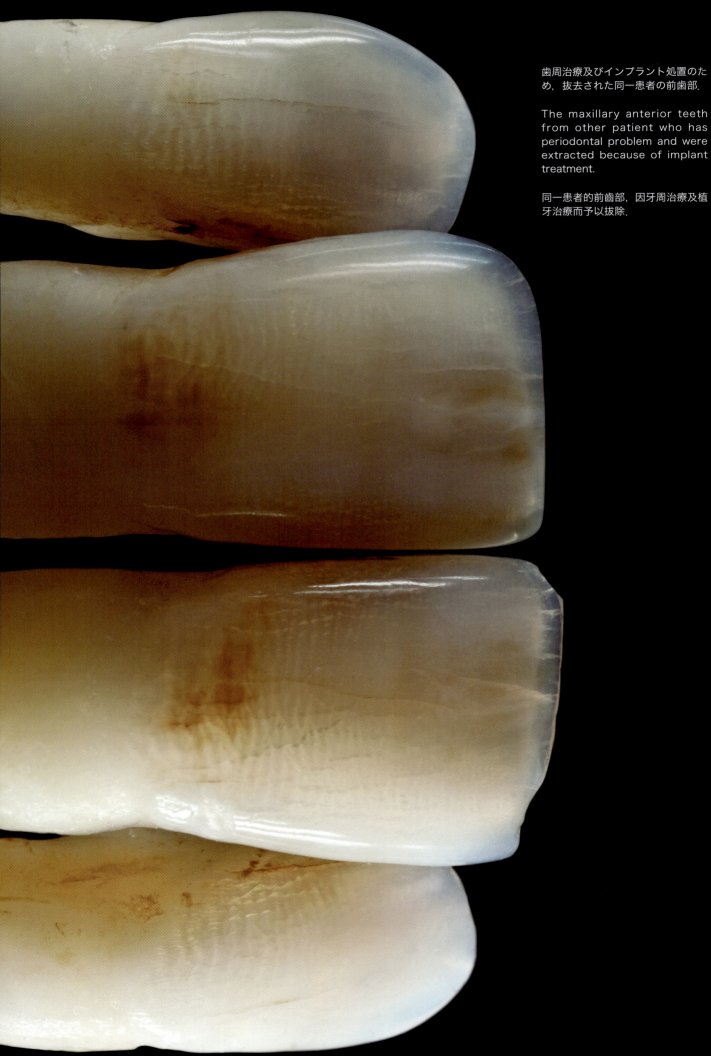

歯周治療及びインプラント処置のため，抜去された同一患者の前歯部．

The maxillary anterior teeth from other patient who has periodontal problem and were extracted because of implant treatment.

同一患者的前齒部，因牙周治療及植牙治療而予以拔除．

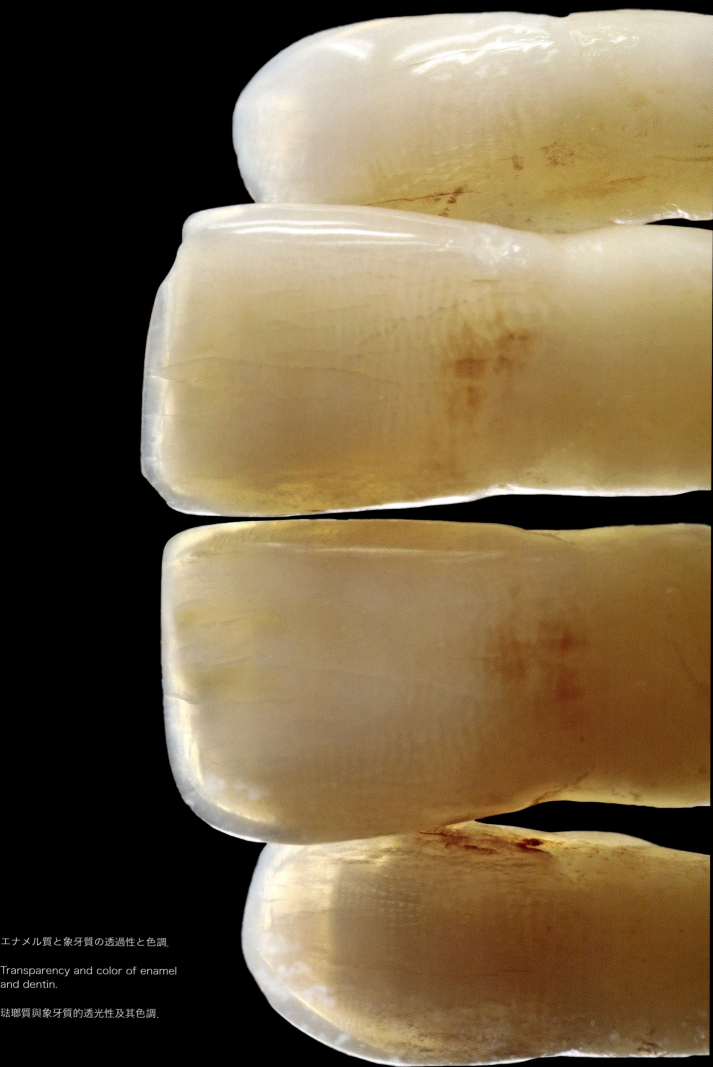

エナメル質と象牙質の透過性と色調.

Transparency and color of enamel and dentin.

琺瑯質與象牙質的透光性及其色調.

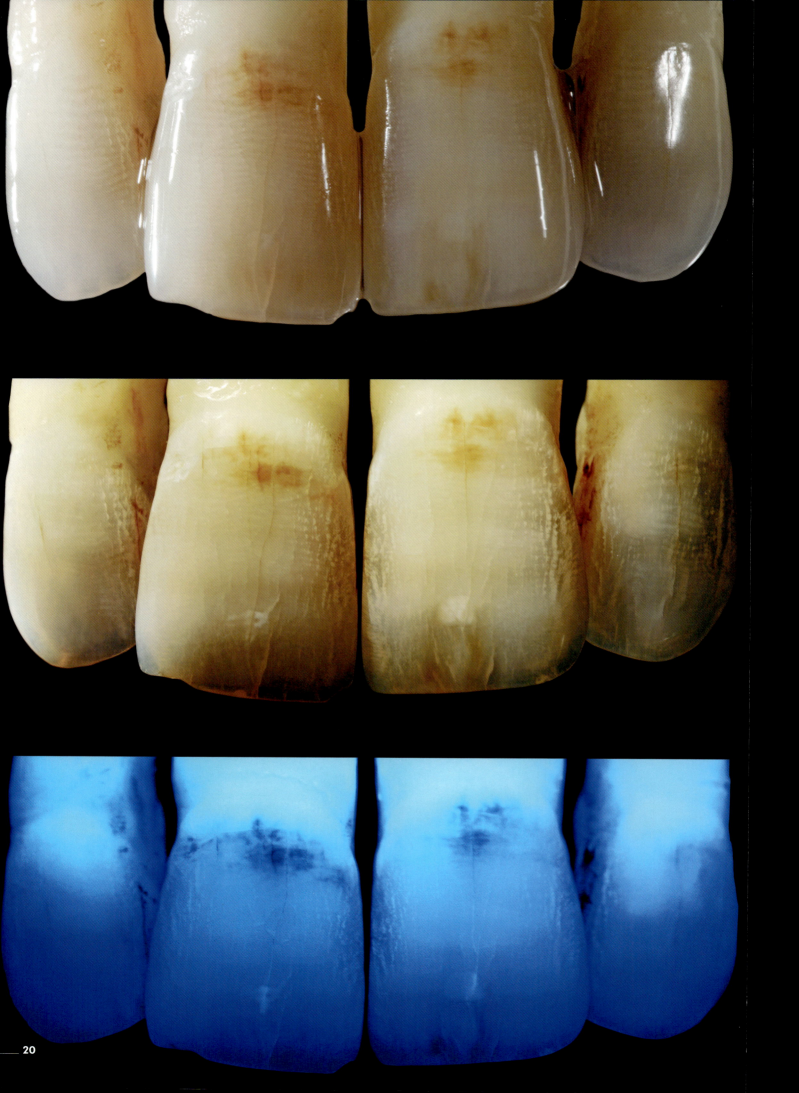

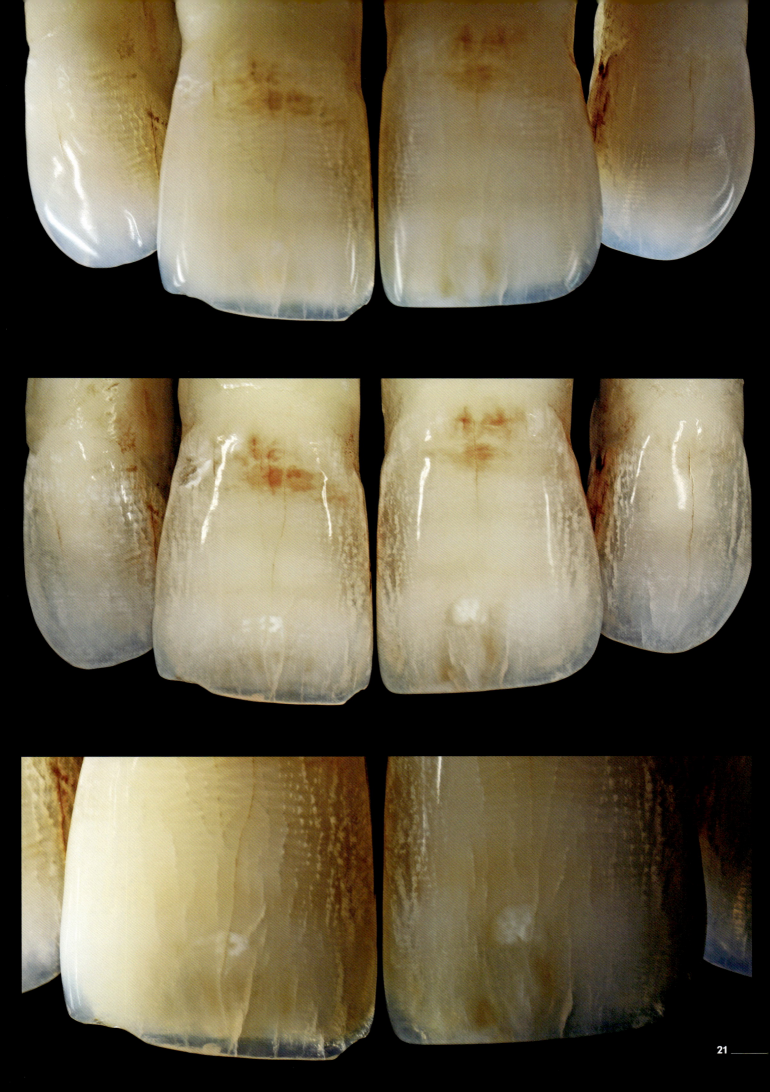

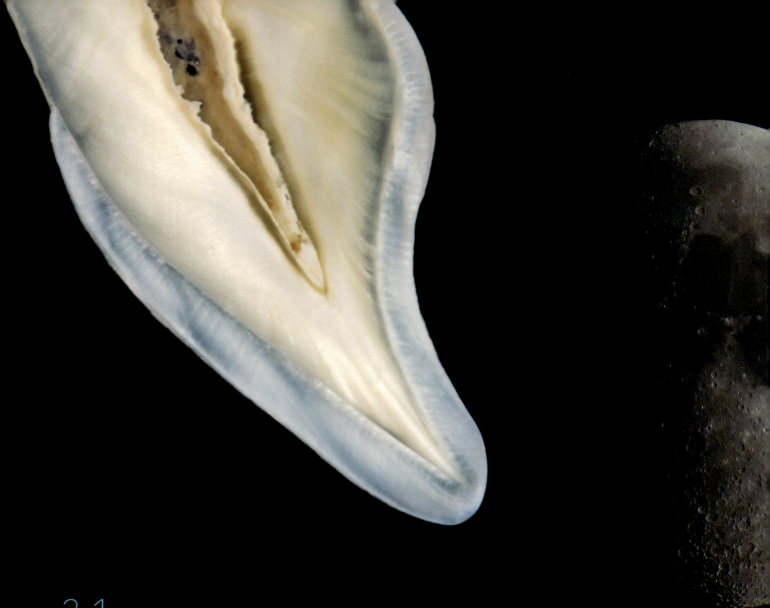

Part 2-1
Internal structure and optical

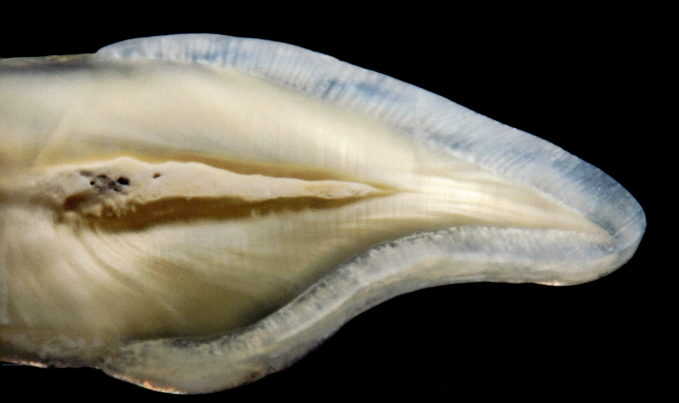

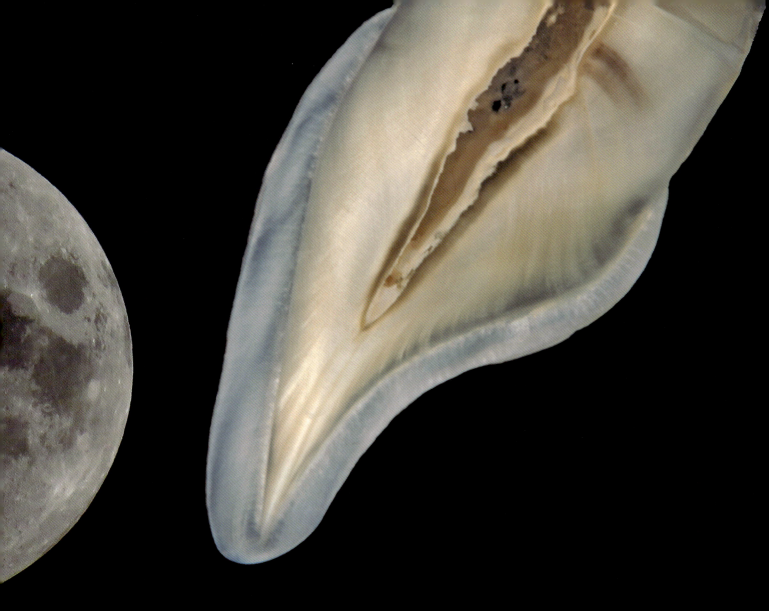

properties of maxillary anterior teeth

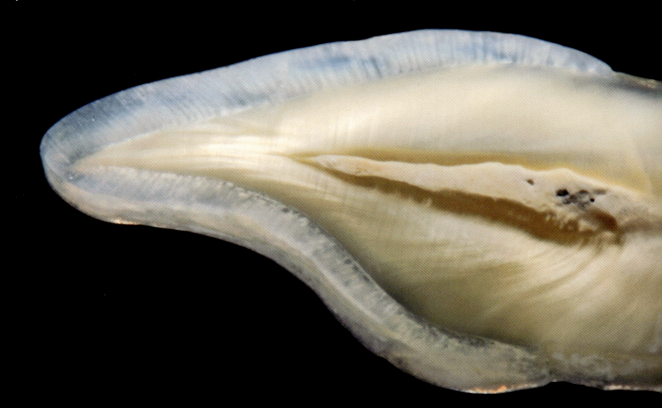

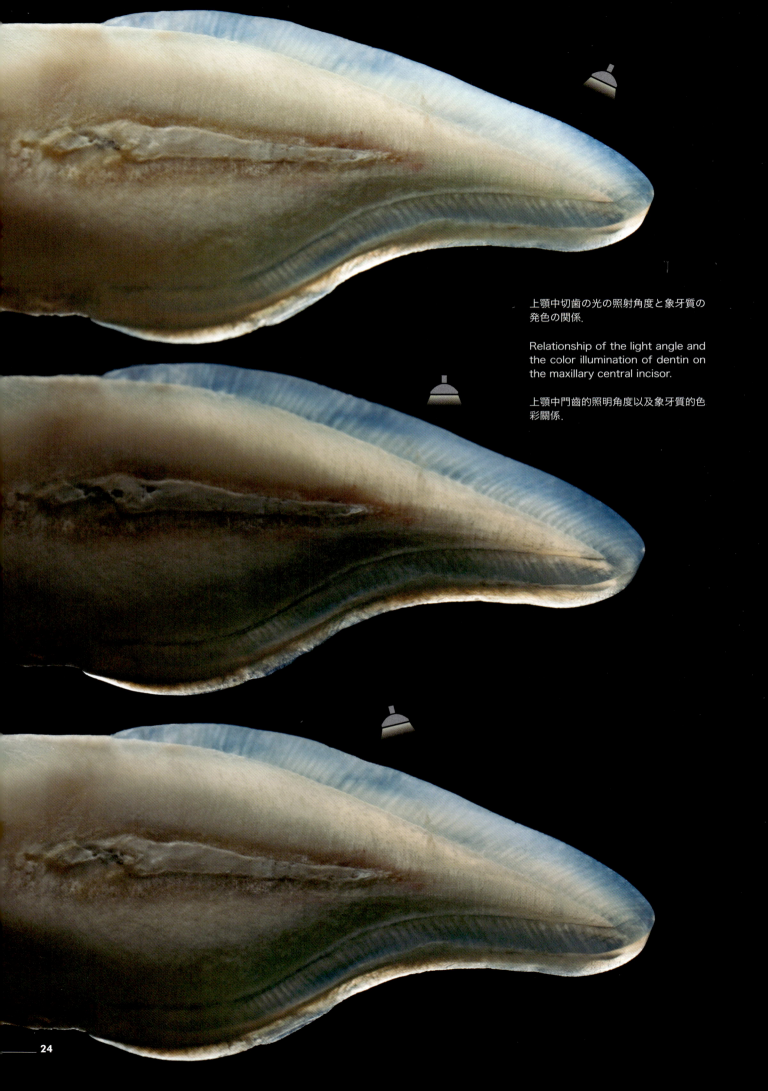

上顎中切歯の光の照射角度と象牙質の発色の関係.

Relationship of the light angle and the color illumination of dentin on the maxillary central incisor.

上顎中門齒的照明角度以及象牙質的色彩關係.

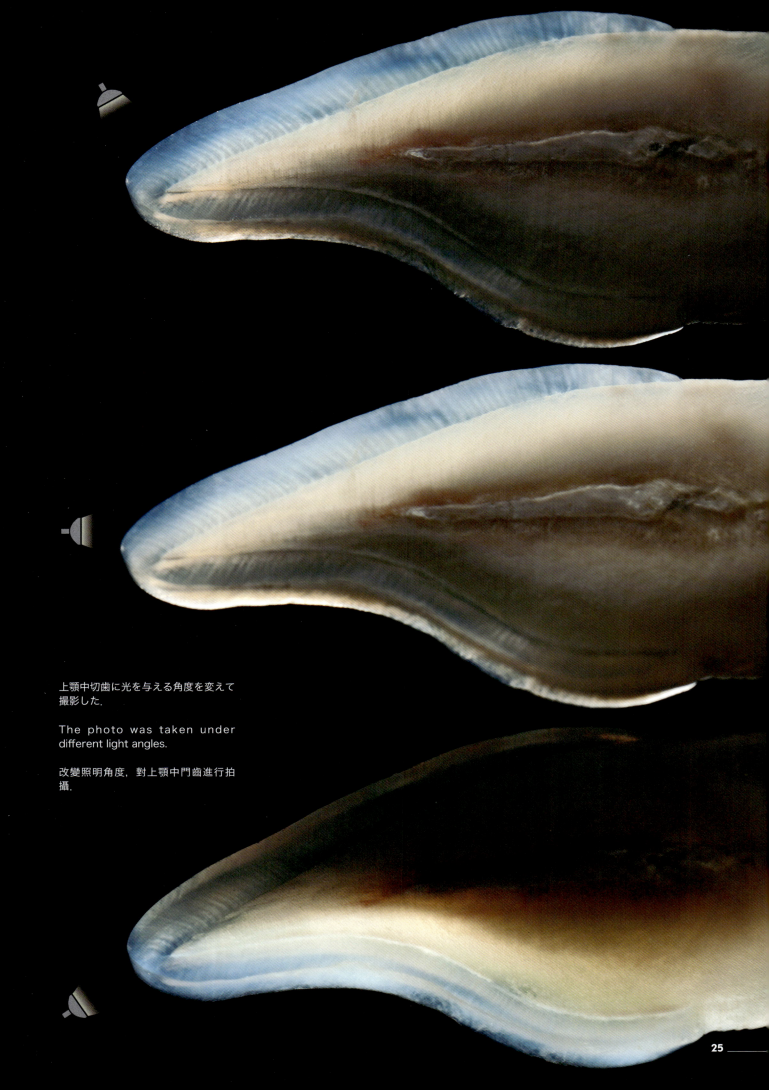

上顎中切歯に光を与える角度を変えて撮影した.

The photo was taken under different light angles.

改變照明角度，對上顎中門齒進行拍攝.

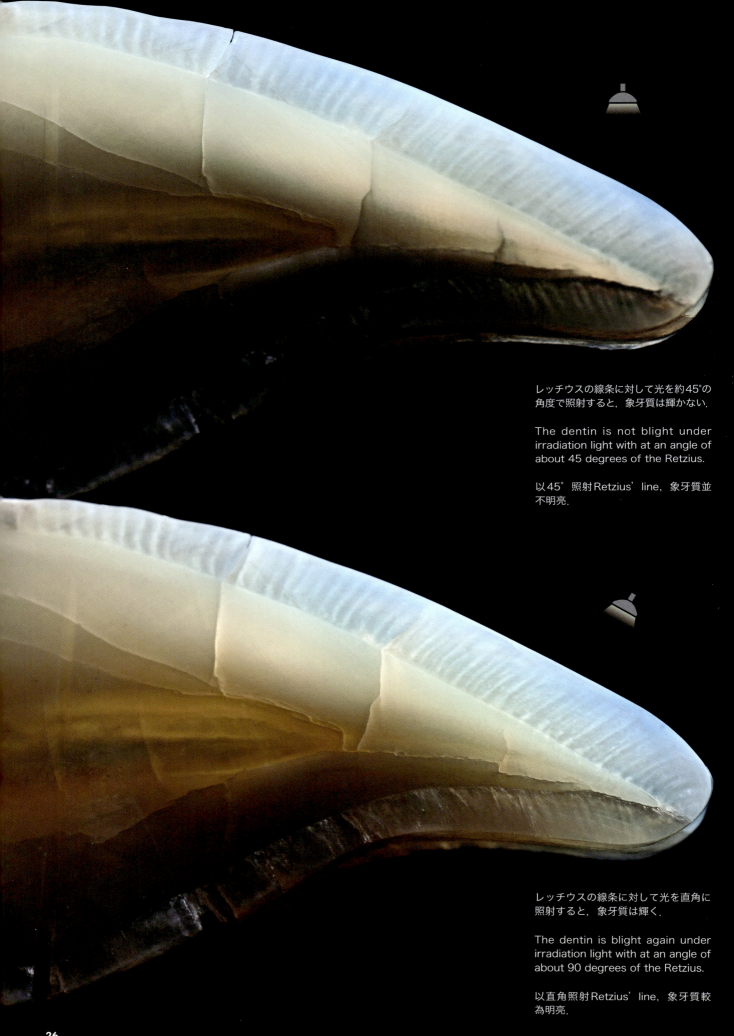

レッチウスの線条に対して光を約45°の角度で照射すると，象牙質は輝かない．

The dentin is not blight under irradiation light with at an angle of about 45 degrees of the Retzius.

以45°照射Retzius'line，象牙質並不明亮．

レッチウスの線条に対して光を直角に照射すると，象牙質は輝く．

The dentin is blight again under irradiation light with at an angle of about 90 degrees of the Retzius.

以直角照射Retzius'line，象牙質較為明亮．

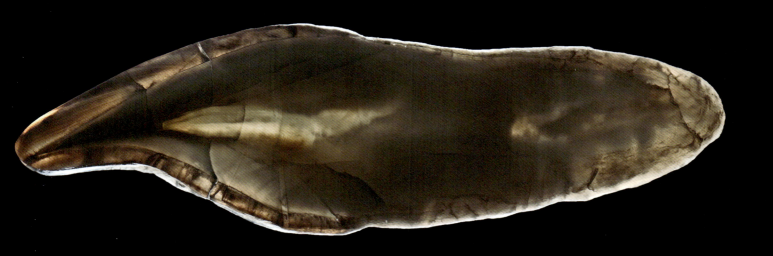

通常，歯は口腔内において歯根にまで届くような光を受けることはないのだが，歯冠に対して人為的に照射された光は象牙質の表面で歯根にまで伝わる．

Normally the light never go through to the root, but under the artificial light, the light pass through the dentin to the root.

一般情況下光並不會直接進到牙根．照射於牙冠上的光會經由象牙質表面傳到牙根．

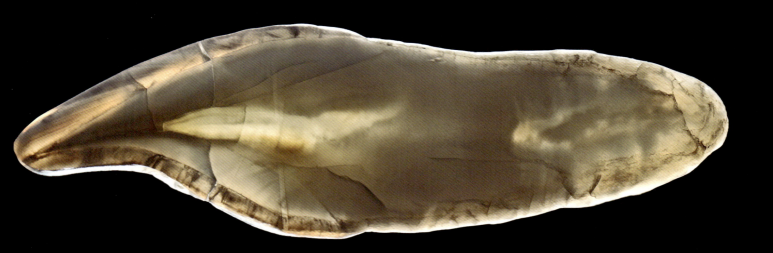

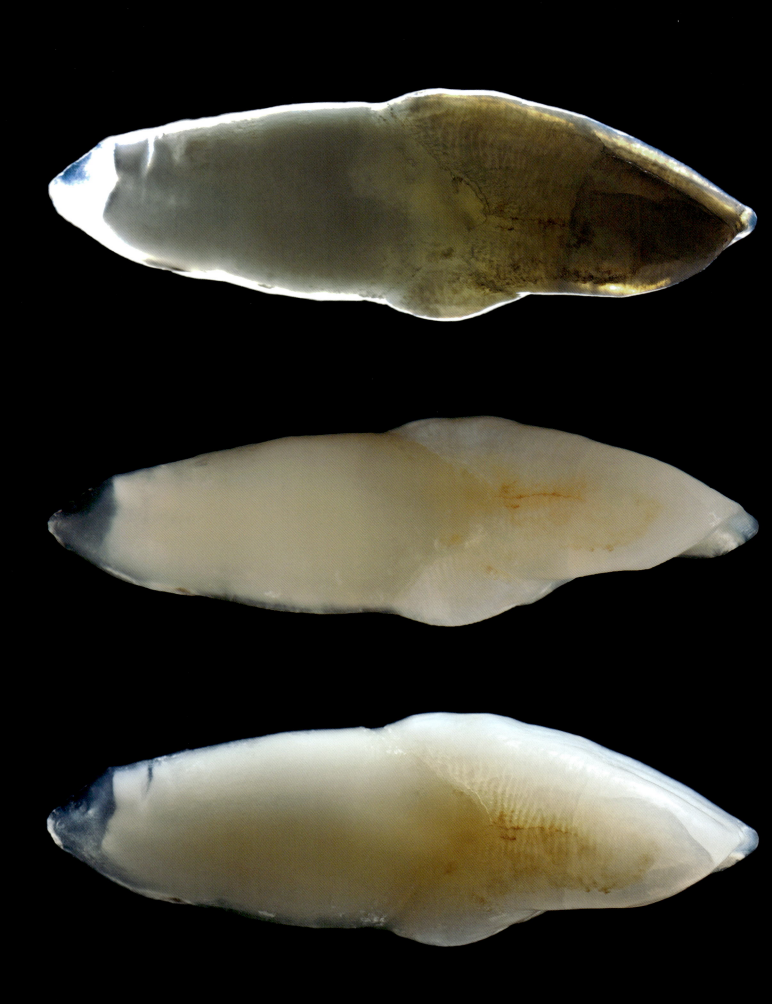

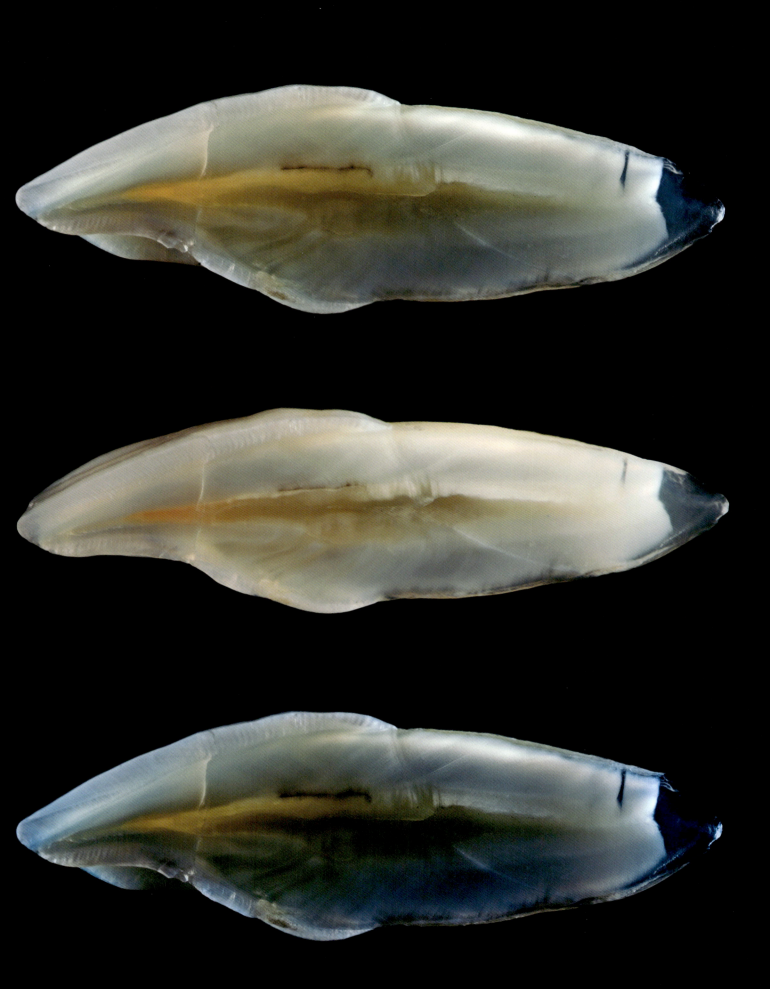

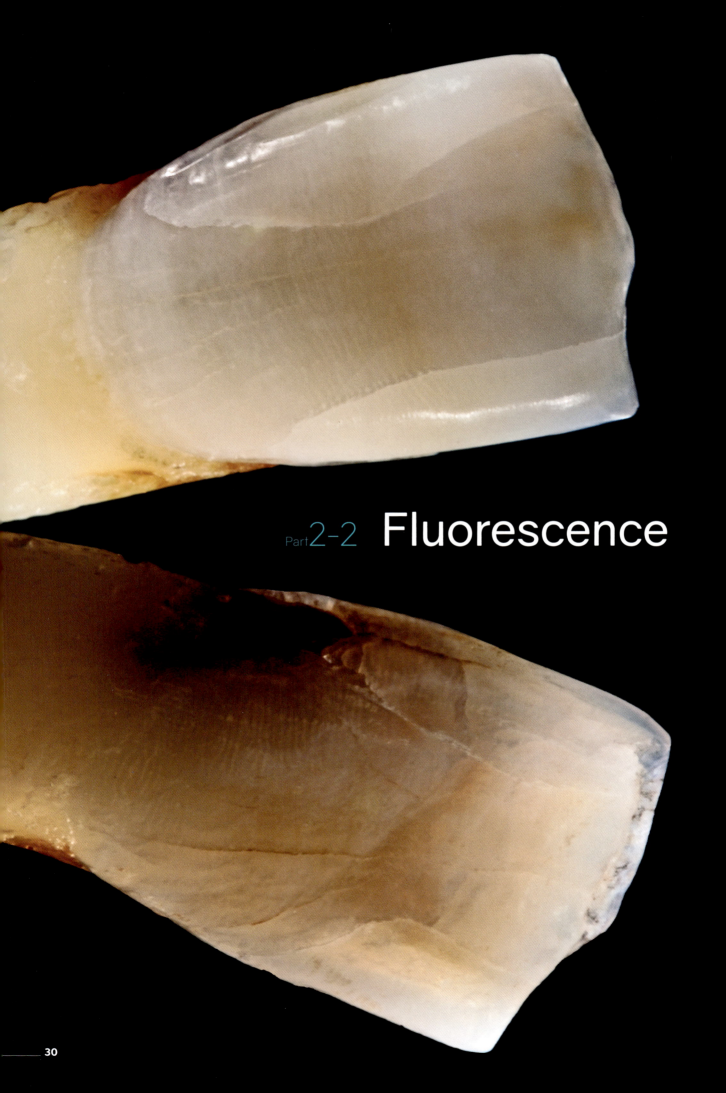

Part 2-2 **Fluorescence**

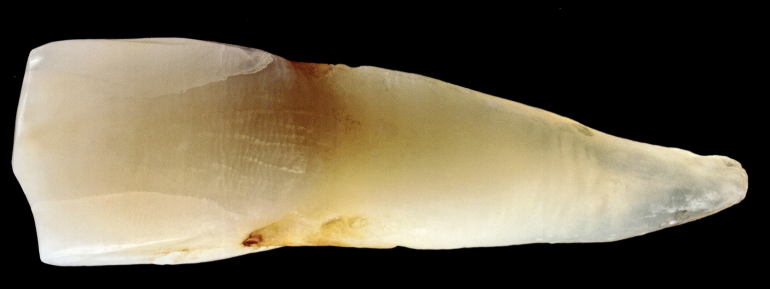

天然歯の蛍光性は色調に大きく影響を及ぼす．

Fluorescence of natural teeth is greatly affecting the color.

天然牙的螢光性質對其色調帶來極大的影響．

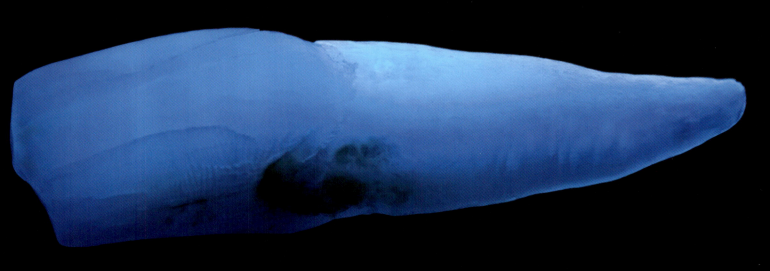

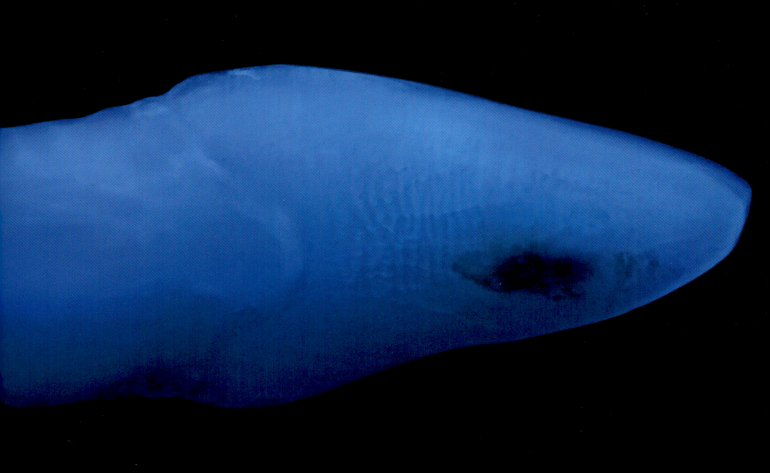

エナメル質には蛍光性は観察できない.

Fluorescence is never observed in the enamel.

琺瑯質上無法觀察到螢光性質.

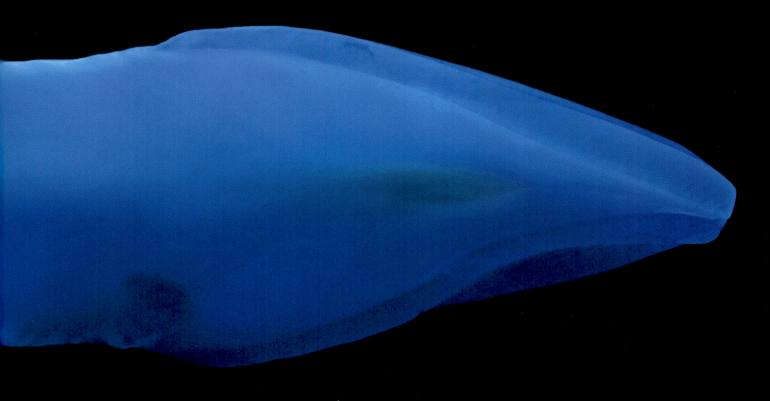

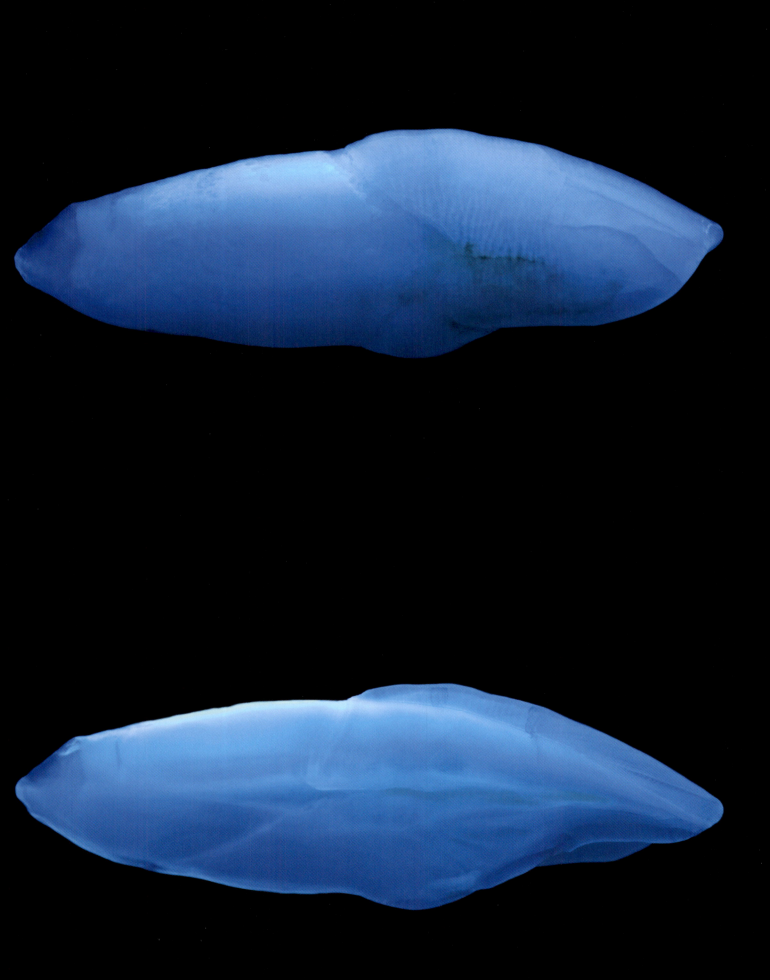

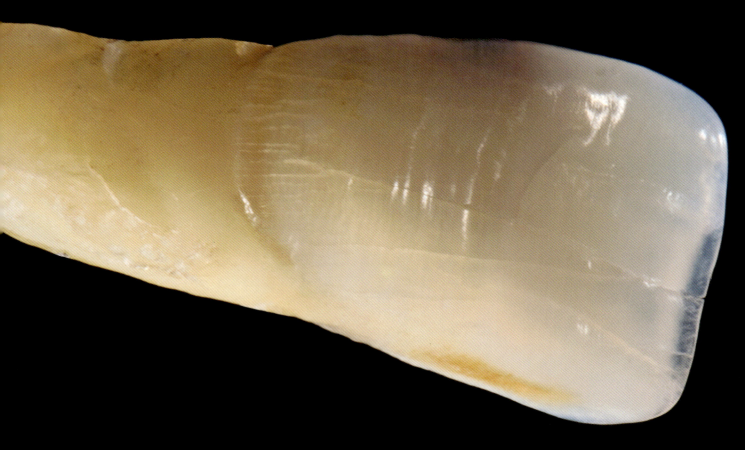

上顎中切歯に摩耗はあるものの，まだ完全な二次象牙質がなく歯髄腔がある歯.

Tooth wear was observed, however there was a pulp without secondary dentin.

有著磨耗的上顎中門齒，以及牙髓腔中並沒有完整的二次象牙質.

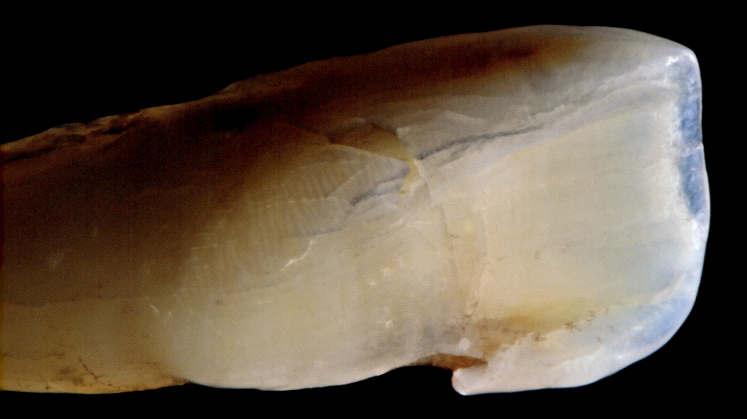

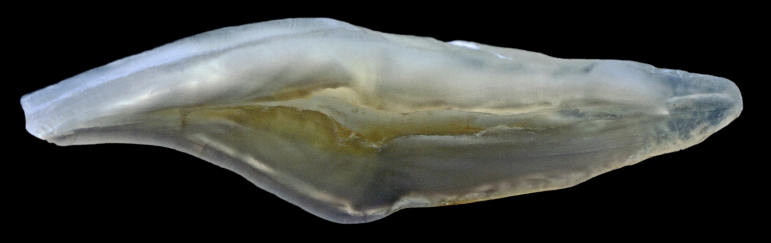

内部に空洞があることにより光が空洞から裏側へと通過しないため,歯髄腔がある前歯部の明度は高く感じられる.

The brightness of an anterior teeth is higher, because the light is never pass through the teeth which has an internal space called as a pulp.

由於內部有空洞,使光無法進到裏層,因此擁有齒髓腔的前齒部明度上會感覺較亮.

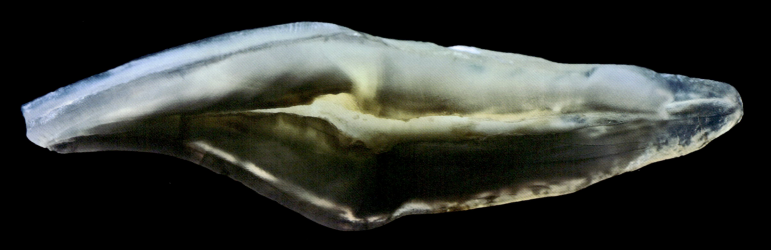

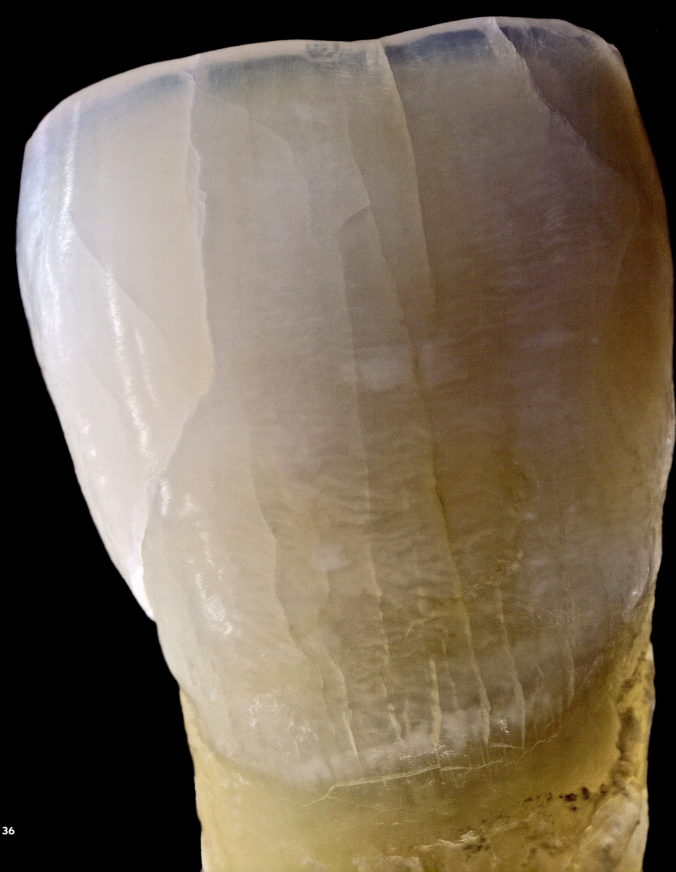

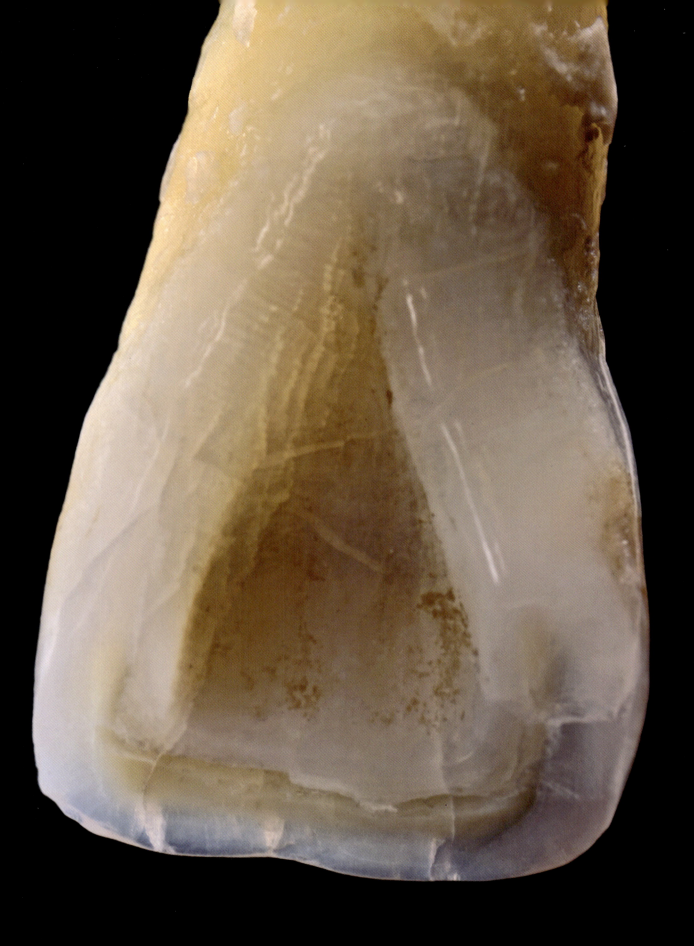

上顎前歯部の内部構造（象牙質）は口蓋側からも観察できる．

Internal structure (dentin) of the maxillary anterior teeth can be observed from the palatal side.

從腭側可觀察到上顎前齒的內部構造（象牙質）．

Part 3

Prologue: Linked to Palatal

The influence of tooth crown colors according to 3 types of internal structure

筆者が陶材による補綴物製作に着手した30余年前，シェードの記録はスケッチで行うことが主流であり，歯科技工士がシェードテイキングに出向かない場合，シェードガイドナンバーやチェアサイドからの簡単な指示のみで作業を行うことも珍しくはなかった．筆者は歯科技工士養成校を卒業後，2軒の院内ラボに通算5年勤務した．その間，日常の業務として患者の口腔内を直接観察し，シェードテイキングや試適，最終補綴物の装着に立ち会うことができた．

その後，セラミックス補綴を主体としたラボを開業するも，色調についてハイレベルな要求が多々舞い込み，再製を余儀なくされることもあった．その原因を考えると，まずは不適切な基本色の付与が挙げられる．ただし，これは筆者の経験と材料知識の不足によるところも大きかった．次に考えられたのが，エナメル質の透明度の不適切な付与である．しかし，単純にエナメル質の透明度

When I started ceramic work more than 30 years before, normally the record of tooth color was taken by illustration. Sometime when I cannot check the tooth color by myself, I worked with very few information as a guide number. I was working five years in dental laboratory at the private practice after graduate two years dental technicians course. I could observe a patient mouth from shade-taking to final procedure. After my office was started, sometime patient was not satisfied my ceramic work, and I needed to re-build. First, the reason why color miss-much was observed, miss-much of base color was happened. The second reason is the miss-mach of the transparency of the enamel. But if internal structure is not fit for the patient characteristic, the result of color much might be worth. Therefore application of the

筆者在三十年前開始製作陶材補綴物時，主要是以素描方式記錄相關shade，一般來說要是沒有外出shade taking，就會從chair side收到簡易指示的Shade guidenumber．筆者從齒科技師養成學校畢業後，五年裡就職過兩間的院內牙技所，日常的業務能夠直接對患者口腔進行直接的觀察，包括直接面對現場shade taking，try in，直到最後的補綴物裝載．之後開業主要以ceramic補綴為主，色調表現均以高標準為目標的前提下，過程中不免一再的重製，在種種考量之後，會先排除不適當的基本色，當然也是因為當時經驗以及材料知識的不足導致，另外也對於琺瑯質透明度的不當呈現．單純只是提高透明度，而沒有付予天然牙洋梨狀的象牙質構造，明顯的呈現出不自然的結果．反而在呈現不透明時，色調在深度上難以表現，為解開此問題點，筆者在這裡以象牙質構造，色調，表面特徵以及型態

Mamelon Type

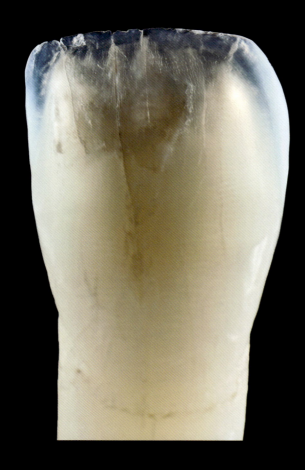
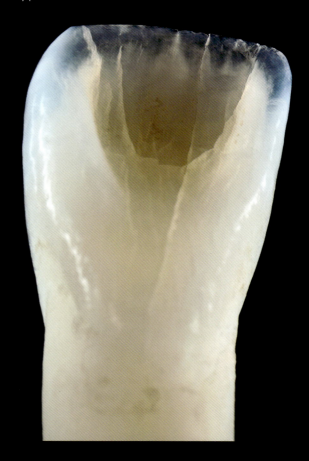

を上げたところで，天然歯のような自然な象牙質（デンティン）構造を適切に再現したり付与できたりしていなければ，不自然さをより際立たせる結果にもなりかねない．だからといって，逆にエナメル質を不透明にすると，色調の深みが表現できない．後者の問題点を解決するために，筆者は本章で示す象牙質の構造と色調及びキャラクター，さらには形態との関連性の考察を開始するに至った．

象 牙質は光を与えなければ，明るくは見えない．光を照射すると，歯頸部が非常に明るくなる他，切縁から約3mm下の象牙質も明るくなっていることが観察できる．そのエリアには，象牙質の構造が最も微細となるマメロン等が観察される．このことを応用して，筆者は直接的あるいは画像等で間接的に観察した天然歯におけるシェード，隣在歯の形態，舌側形態を20年以上にわたって観察，記録してきた．これらを分析すると，前述したように内部構造と歯冠色，形態に相関性が見られたのである．

transparency of an enamel is very important, and the relationship in between these of dentin structure, color balance and morphology. So I was started observation.

Dentin cannot be seen without the light. Under the light, cervical and the area 2 mm from the incisal edge start blighting. In that area, the structure of dentin is very complicate, observed as a mamelon. I collected directly and/or indirectly as a photo observation of natural teeth color and morphology based on this idea for more than 20 years. When analyzed these datas, the correlation between internal structure, crown color and shape of tooth structure was observed.

上的關聯性來進行說明．

若 不賦予象牙質光線，便無法看到它的明暗．由於光的照射，齒頸部變得非常明亮外，切緣下約3mm的象牙質可觀察到一樣明亮的情況，這個區域裡象牙質構造非常地細微，也可以觀察到它的Mamelon型態．筆者經過二十年以上直接觀察或是以圖像間接觀察天然牙的shade．

鄰 牙型態，舌側型態，並予以記錄分析．經過分析可以了解到前述所提到的內部構造和牙冠色以及型態的相關性．

Devil Head M Type

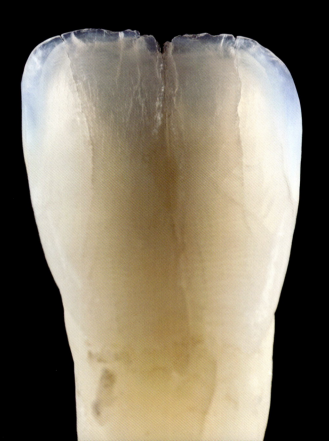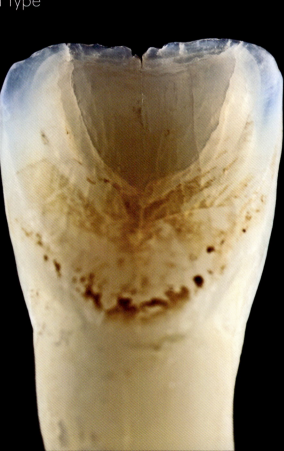

内部構造について見ると，① マメロンが著明なもの（指状構造を呈するもの），② 歯冠形態の縮小型となっているもの，③ 近遠心の隆線部から弓状に灰色の象牙質が観察できるもの（このタイプはさらに① マメロン，② 歯冠の縮小の２種類に分類される），そして④ 非常に形態のテーパーが強く透明感の部位が近遠心部位に強く感じられるもの，に大別された．実際の症例ではこれらの複合型や，さらに例外型として，象牙質とエナメル質の色調が上下で極端に異なっているもの，切縁部の摩耗による象牙質の石灰化から内部構造が変化してマメロンと灰色の象牙質が共存するもの，歯の発育中に薬品による影響でエナメル質が赤変，褐色変しているもの，①と③及び②と④混合型等があるのだが，大きな傾向としては前述の類型に収まっていた（なお，この内部構造の違いは性別ご

With regard to the internal structure, (① shape of mamelon (finger-shape structure)) (② anatomical type) (③ A gray dentin was observed from the mesio-distal ridge. In this type, there are two type of shape, ① Mamelon type ② anatomical type) and (④ very strong taper, and high translucency in the mesio-distal area). Those 4 different types of inside structure were observed. In clinical cases, complex type like combination with ① and ③ or ② and ④ were seen, but mostly include into 4 different types. Sometimes, unusual type were observed like big different tooth color from edge to cervical, combination of mamelon and glay dentin with tooth wear. (In my mind, gender difference was observed. Still this idea is under consideration, but normally mamelon type is more observed in female, because tooth contraction was earlier than male, and also occluding force might be affected.) Additionally, while in tooth growth, drag affect to

關於內部構造可以觀察到，① 有明顯Mamelon指狀構造的部份，② 縮小型牙冠的部份，③ 近遠心隆線有弓形灰色象牙質的部份，這部份又加以分出Mamelon和牙冠縮小型，④ 近遠心有強烈錐型透明感的部份．實際案例上也有複合型或例外的，像是象牙質和琺瑯質的色調有著極端差異的，或者是由於切緣磨耗產生的石灰化所造成Mamelon與灰色象牙質共存現象，也有相對少數的①③混合型，②④混合．筆者同時認為內部構造多少與性別相關，女性永久齒相對較早萌發，或有遺傳，咬合力等種種因素．筆者撰寫本書時尚

Box Type

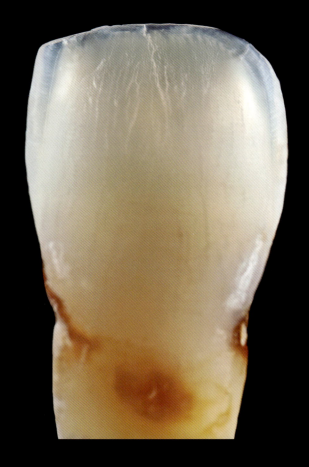
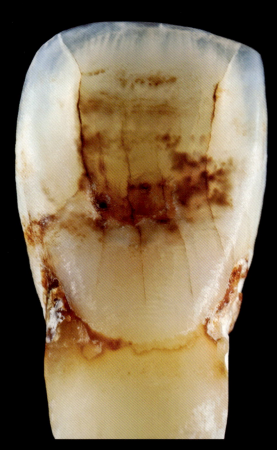

とに若干の違いがあるように筆者は考えている．男性に比べて女性のほうが永久歯に生え変わる時期が早いことや，遺伝，咬合力等，様々な要因によるものと推測でき，本書執筆時点で確たる検証は行えないが，一般的に多く見られるものは，マメロンタイプで，特に女性に多いと感じられる）．

　そこで筆者は，これらの定義に対して，①を「マメロンタイプ（Mamelon Type）」，②を「ボックスタイプ（Box Type）」，③を「デビルヘッドMタイプ（Devil Head M Type）」「デビルヘッドBタイプ（Devil Head B Type）」，④を「テーパータイプ（Taper Type）」との呼称を与えることにした．以下，それぞれの類型における歯の特徴を抜去歯の撮影により示す．

change the tooth color as a red sift or brownies. Therefore, in order to understand easily, those 4 types of typical color was categorized, ① Mamelon type ② Box type ③ Devil head M type and Devil head B type ④ Taper type, Typical samples of those 4 different types are shown below.
Mamelon Type
Devil Head M Type
Box Type
Devil Head B Type

未明確檢證，一般來說女性常見到Mamelon type．附帶一提，在發育中的牙齒也會受藥物影響而變紅變黃．

　這裡筆者為了進行shade taking和shade making，進而將上述概括命名為①Mamelon型②Box型③Devil Head M型，Devil Head B型④Taper型．

Devil Head B Type

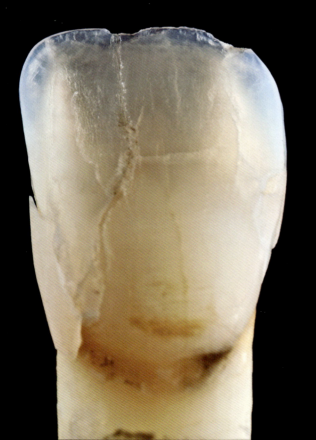
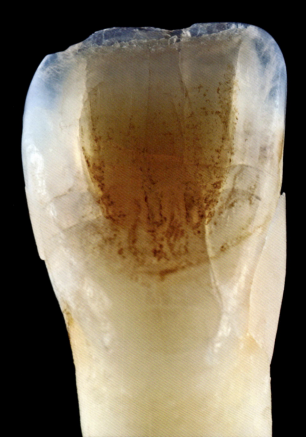

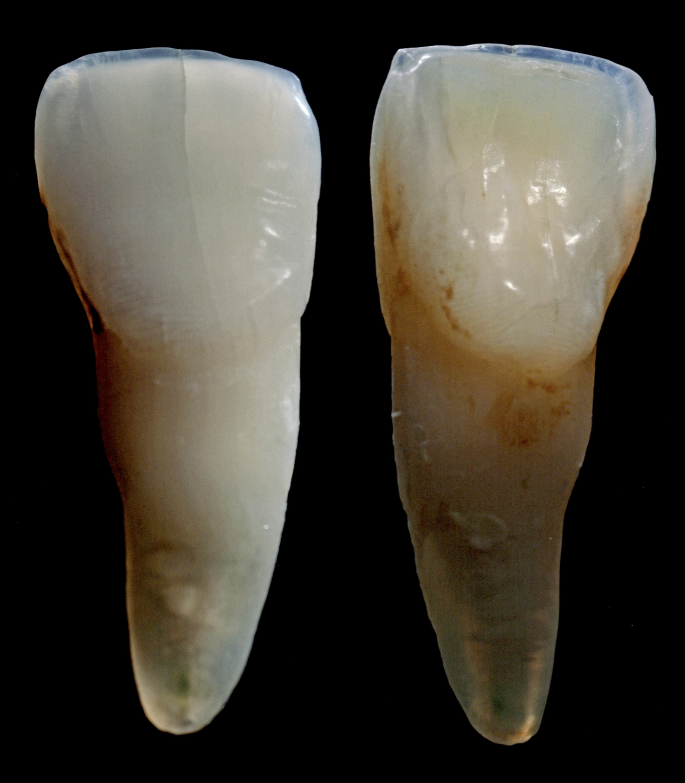

エナメル質の存在により，前歯部の内部構造の観察は容易ではない．歯はエナメル質の厚さと光学特性により一見シンプルに見えるが，その内部にある象牙質の構造及び色調は，複雑な組織により構成されている．

It is not easy to observe the internal structure of anterior teeth, because of outer structure enamel. Of course, the color construction of teeth is very complex affected by light properties, thickness of enamel.

前齒內部構造因為琺瑯質的存在而難以觀察，當然也是有乍看單純的琺瑯質厚度、光學特性，而象牙質構造、色調是複雜的組織構成。

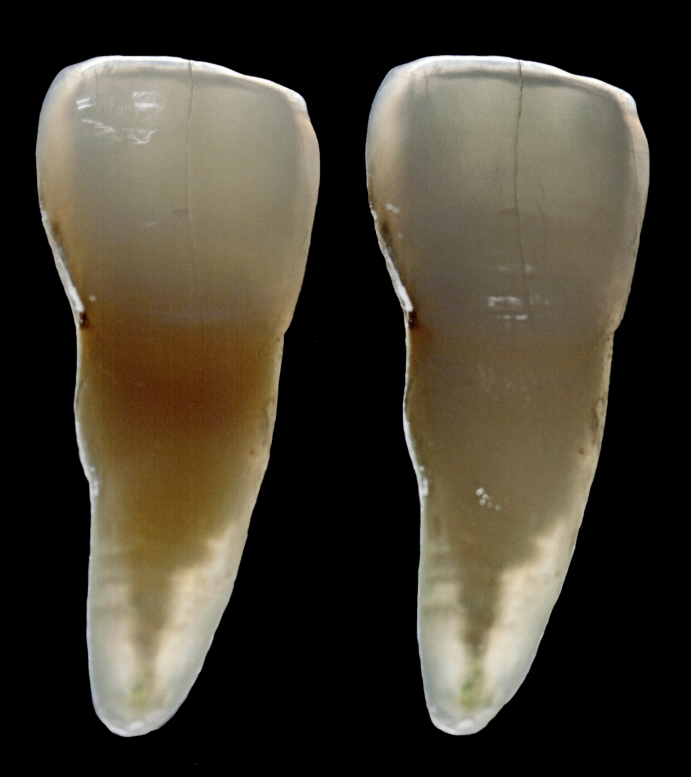

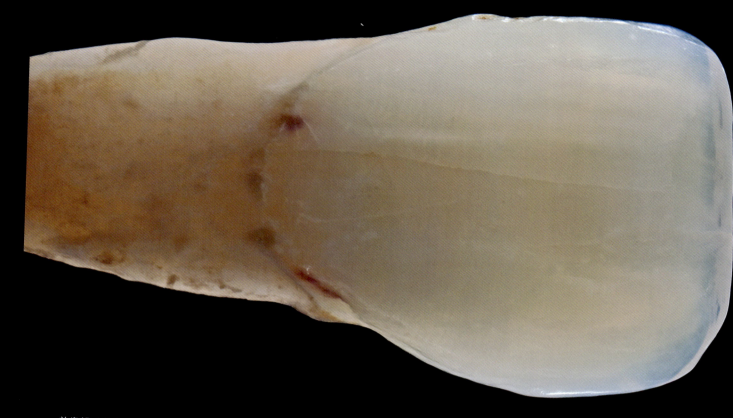

前歯部天然歯の内部構造の見え方は，エナメル質の光学特性と厚さにより影響を受けている．同様に歯冠色の見え方も影響を受けている．

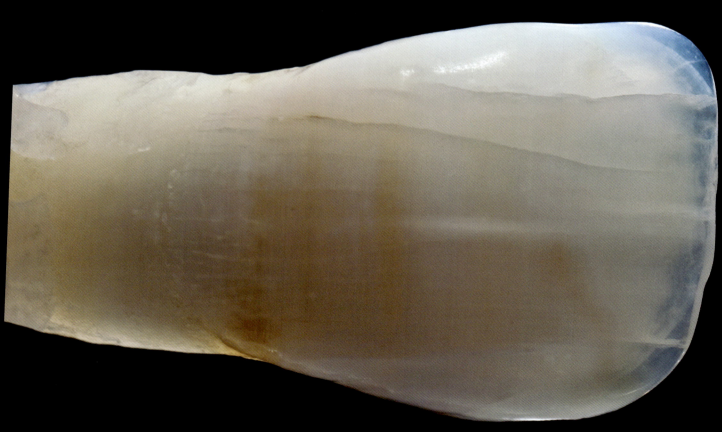

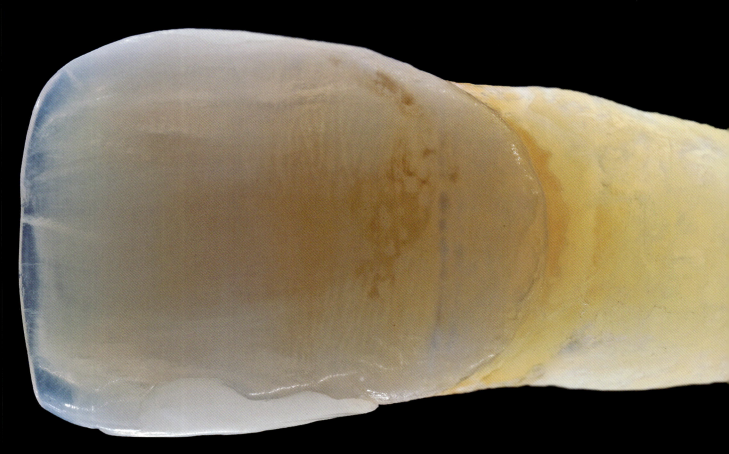

Actuarial color of the anterior teeth is constructed by internal structure and the thickness of an enamel.

前齒的內部構造依據看的方法不同，主要是琺瑯質的光學特性和厚度影響著牙冠的色彩.

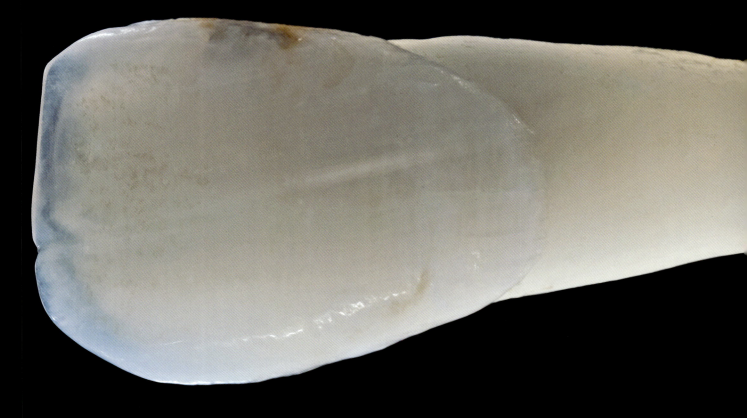

Part 3-1
Mamelon Type

マメロンタイプの歯の特徴として、主に近遠心の隆線が著明であり、中央隆線の形がマメロンの中央部の見え方に連動している。切縁部から観察すると、中央のマメロンは歯冠中央よりもやや遠心に位置している。マメロンの構造を観察すると、縦の繊維状の集合体であることがわかる。マメロンの縁端から1〜2mmほど下に最も明るい部位が存在する。近心と遠心とでは遠心の透明なエリアの幅が広くなっている。

Characteristic of Mamelon type, normally medial and distal ridge are remarkable, and central ridge is related with the view of center part of Mamelon. The observation from an incisal edge, center part of Mamelon is located distal side. Structure of Mamelon is shown like bundle of fibers directed to vertical direction. Brightest area is observed 2 mm under the edge of Mamelon. The transparent are of distal side is wider then medial side.

Mamelon型的特徵主要是近遠心隆線較為明顯，觀察中央Mamelon的視點盡而影響中間隆線的型態。從切緣可觀察到中間的Mamelon略為偏遠心。觀察Mamelon的構造，可看到縱向的纖維群。從Mamelon切緣端下1〜2mm是最為明亮的部份。另外，遠心的透明區域是比較廣的。

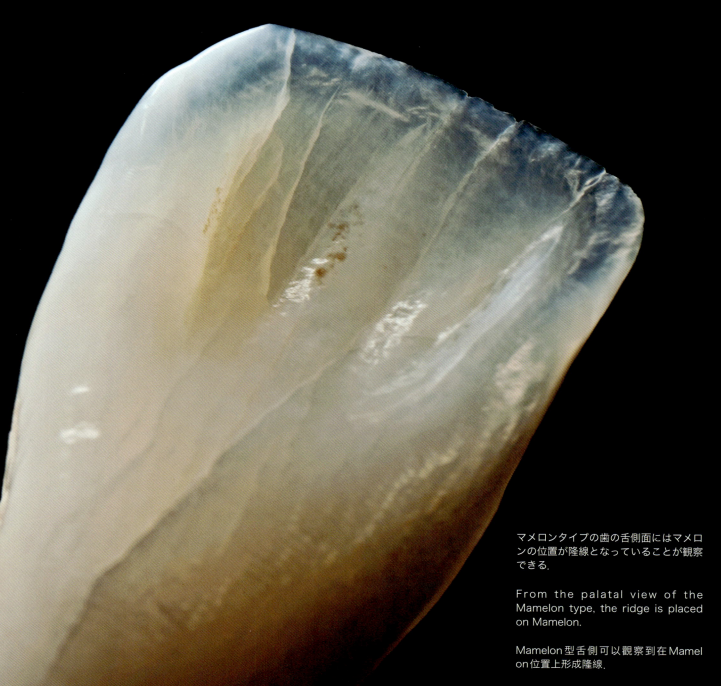

マメロンタイプの歯の舌側面にはマメロンの位置が隆線となっていることが観察できる。

From the palatal view of the Mamelon type, the ridge is placed on Mamelon.

Mamelon型舌側可以觀察到在Mamelon位置上形成隆線。

筆者がマメロンタイプの歯の色調再現を行う場合は，マメロンの谷間には蛍光性を持たないオリーブグリーンの陶材を使用している．マメロン部のバックにはオパール効果のある陶材でマメロン部の縁端を囲んでいる．

My technique of construction on Mamelon type, olive green porcelain without fluorescence is used in between the Mamelon. In addition, opal effected porcelain is placed surrounding the edge of the Mamelon.

筆者在表現Mamelon型時，會在Mamelon谷間使用不具有螢光性的olive green陶材．

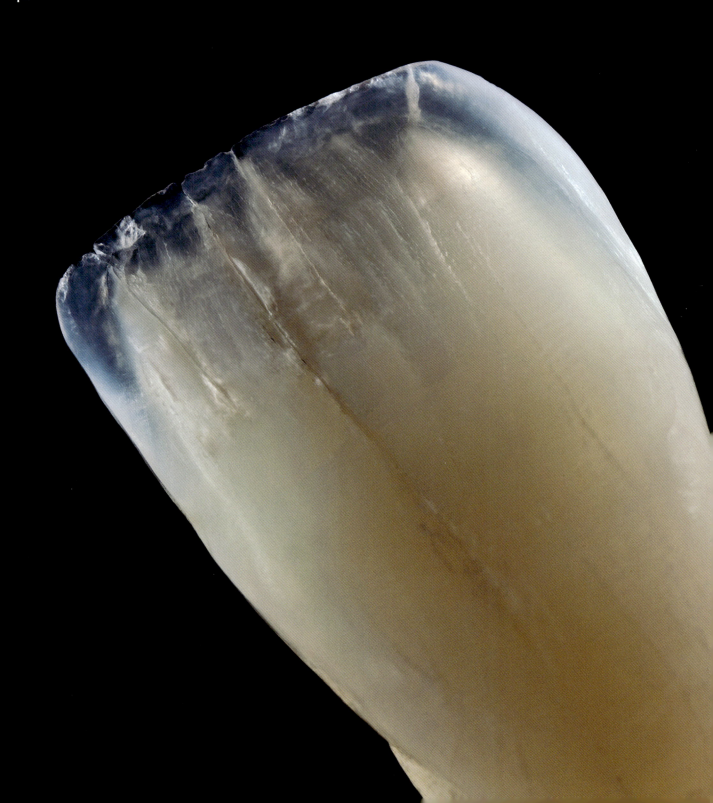

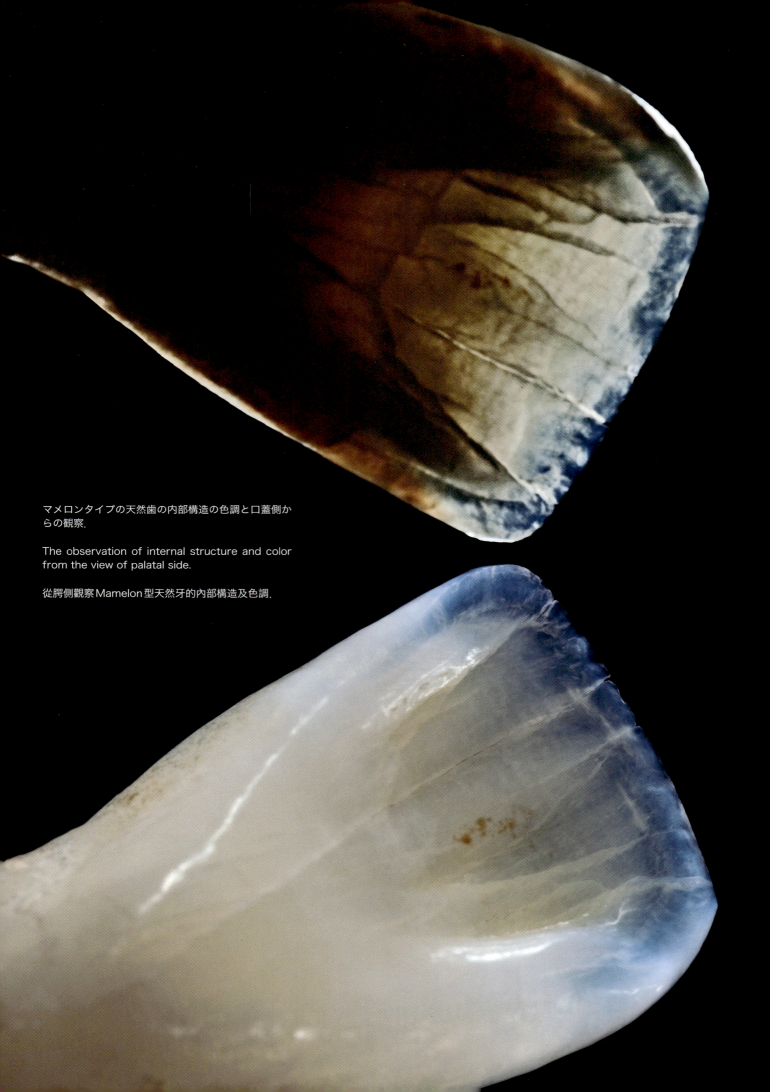

マメロンタイプの天然歯の内部構造の色調と口蓋側からの観察.

The observation of internal structure and color from the view of palatal side.

從腭側觀察Mamelon型天然牙的內部構造及色調.

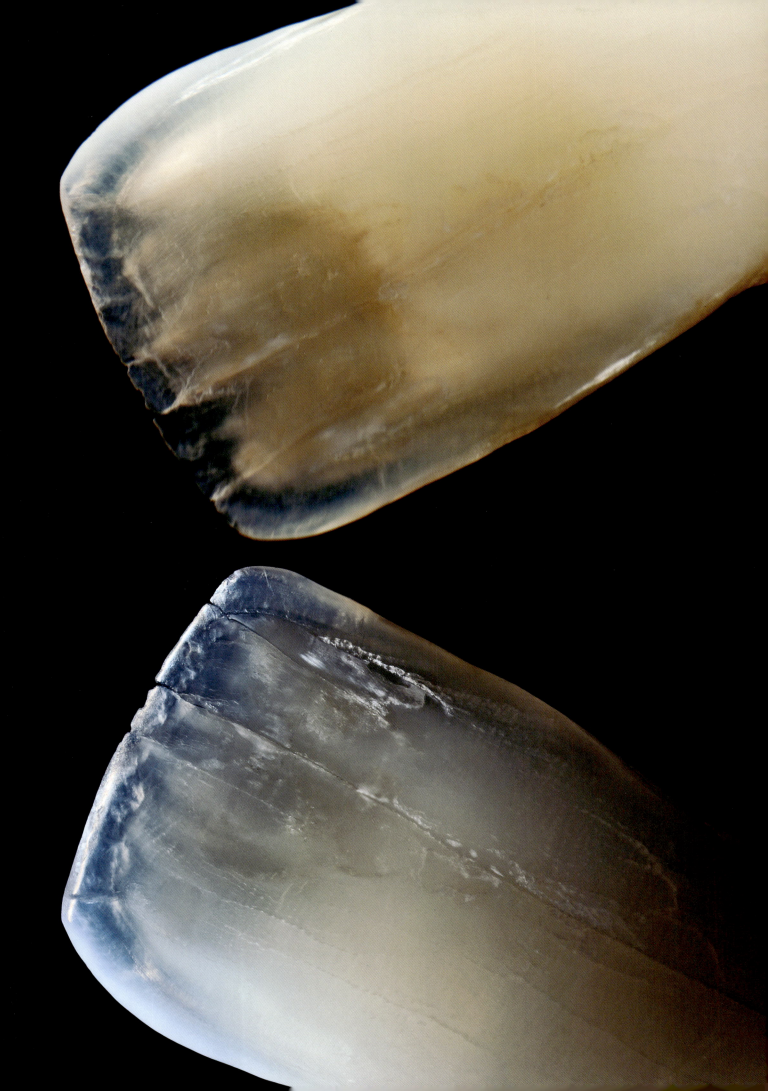

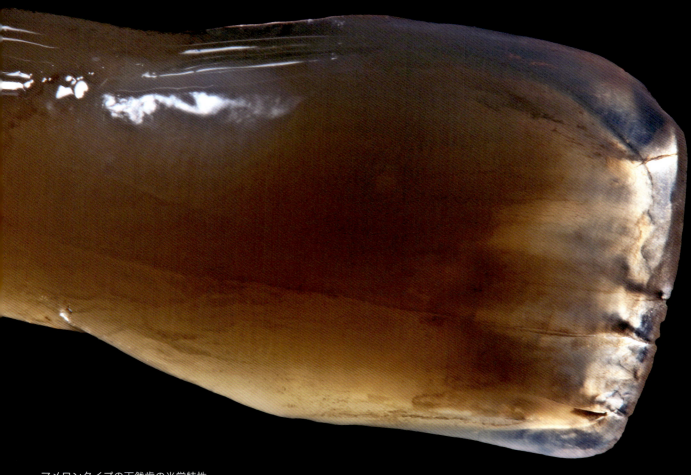

マメロンタイプの天然歯の光学特性.
近遠心の縦に伸びた構造と歯冠中央部の縦の構造とが
著明に観察できる.

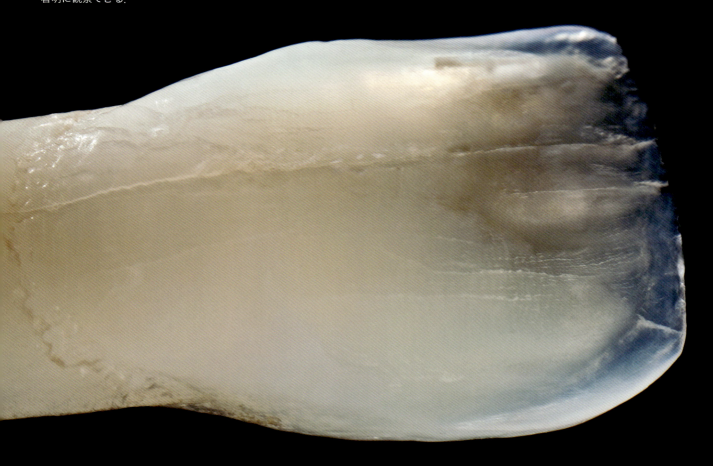

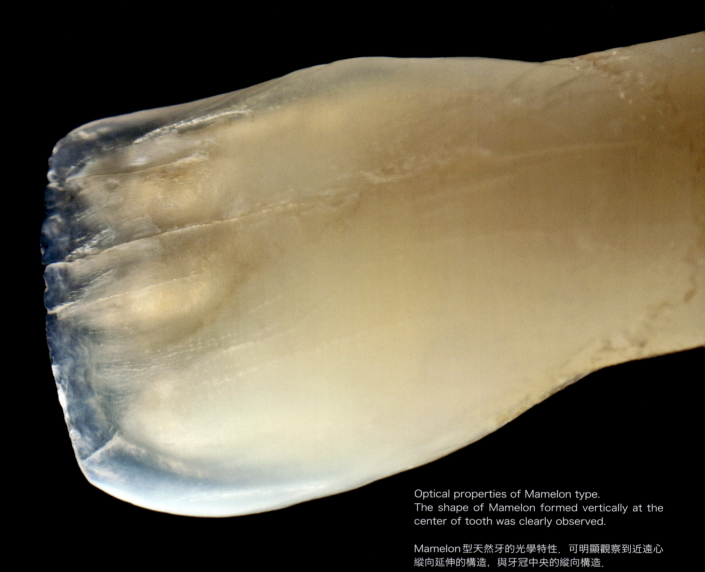

Optical properties of Mamelon type.
The shape of Mamelon formed vertically at the center of tooth was clearly observed.

Mamelon型天然牙的光學特性,可明顯觀察到近遠心縱向延伸的構造,與牙冠中央的縱向構造.

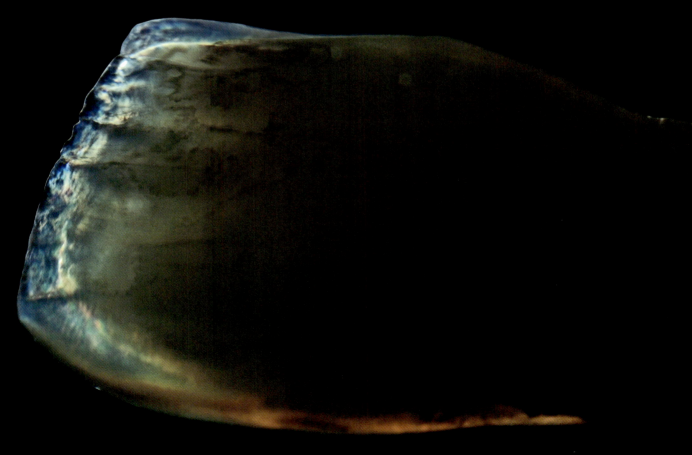

マメロンタイプの天然歯の構造.
歯冠中央部と近遠心の縦に大きく伸びた構造の谷間は，彩度が高く明度は低い．内部構造とエナメル質との境界部にオパール効果が観察できる．

Structure of Mamelon type on the natural teeth.
High brightness area without clarity was observed between the Mamelon formed vertically at the center of tooth, and, opal effect can be observed between the internal structure and enamel.

Mamelon型天然牙結構.
牙冠中央部和近遠心縱向延伸之間的構造，有彩度上的呈現，並無明度呈現，內部構造及琺瑯質交界可觀察到opal.

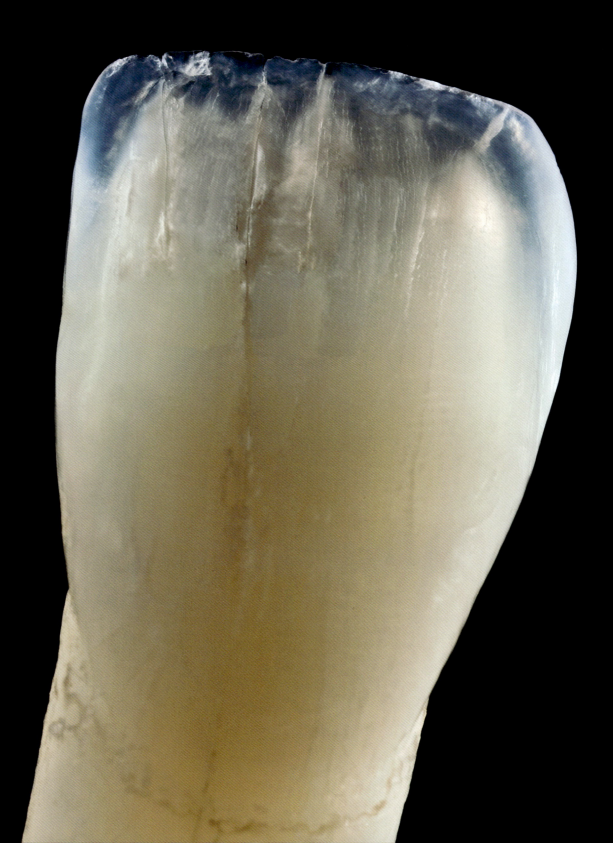

切縁に摩耗が観察できないマメロンタイプの天然歯では，象牙質の内部に明度の高い構造が見られる．よって若年層のマメロンタイプの歯の象牙質は，透過光下では不透明である．

In the Mamelon type without tooth wear at the incisal edge, high brightness area was clearly observed. Thus in younger age, Mamelon type shows opaque under the transmitted light.

切緣沒有磨耗的Mamelon型天然牙，象牙質內部構造可觀察到有較高的明度，因此年輕族群所呈現的Mamelon型，象牙質在透過光照射下所呈現的是不透明的．

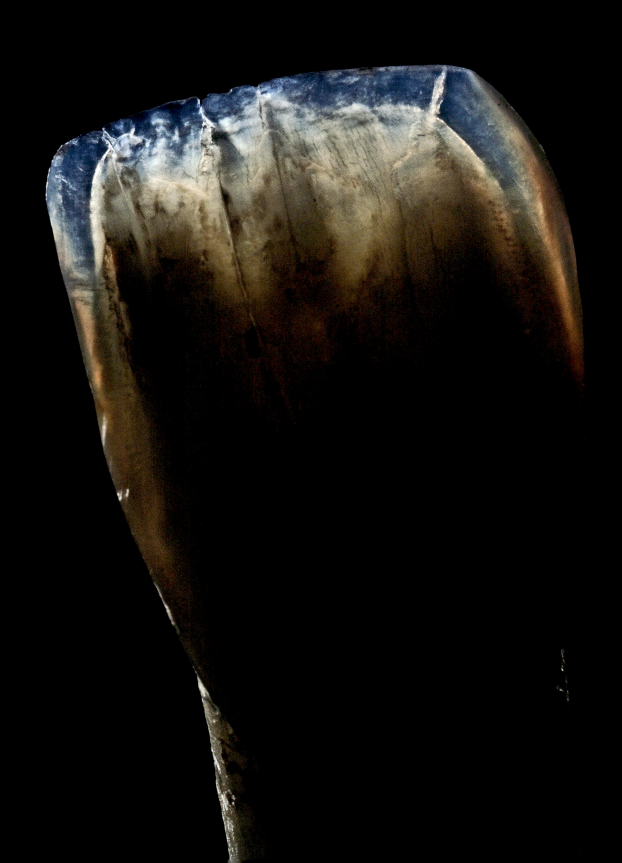

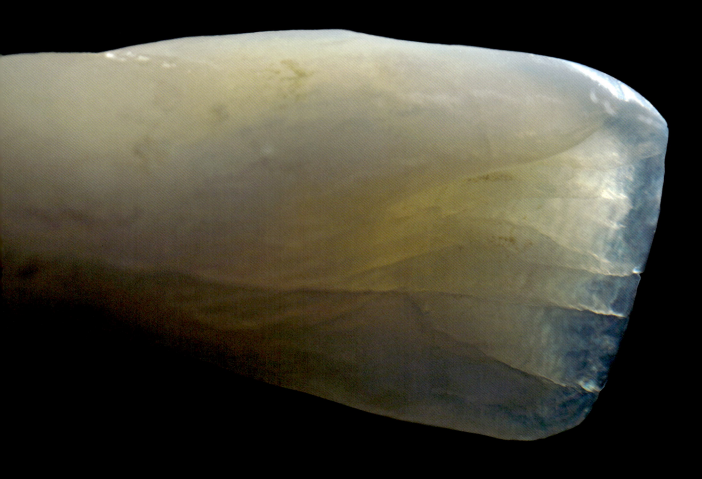

マメロンタイプの歯の口蓋側からの観察.
マメロン構造は口蓋側からも観察できる.エナメル質
は唇側よりも薄いため透過光ではエナメル質の波状の
光学特性が観察できる.

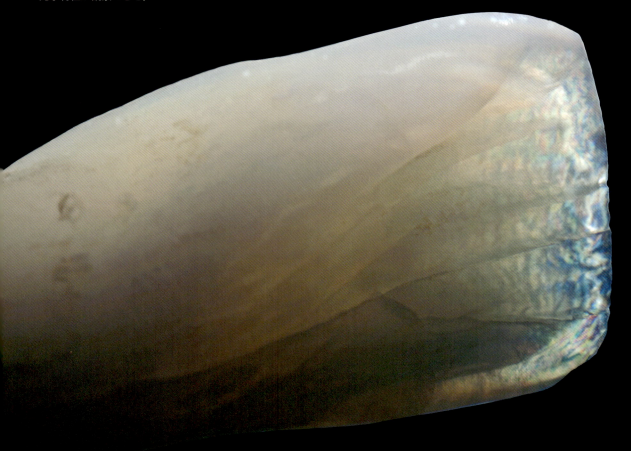

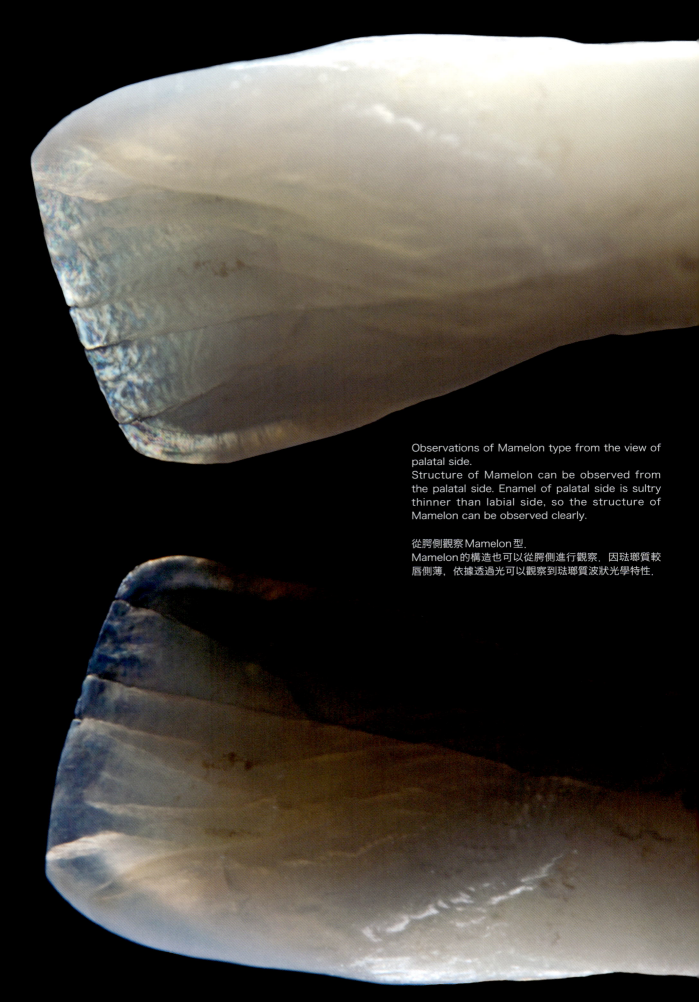

Observations of Mamelon type from the view of palatal side.
Structure of Mamelon can be observed from the palatal side. Enamel of palatal side is sultry thinner than labial side, so the structure of Mamelon can be observed clearly.

從腭側觀察Mamelon型.
Mamelon的構造也可以從腭側進行觀察. 因琺瑯質較唇側薄, 依據透過光可以觀察到琺瑯質波狀光學特性.

Part 3-2
Mamelon Type + Box Type

マメロンタイプとボックスタイプの中間的な歯もある．この歯の特徴として，マメロンの本数が概ね5本程度あり，マメロンの大きさが遠心で最も大きく，次に近心のマメロン，そして中央部のマメロンは細いものが3〜5本程度観察できる．近遠心の隅角

Intermediate type between the Mamelon type and box type is also observed. Characteristic of Intermediate type, normally there are five peaks of Mamelon. Distal Mamelon is the largest and medial Mamelon is second large. In

介於Mamelon型和Box型之間的天然牙．此天然牙的特徵是Mamelon會出現5束，遠心的Mamelon範圍會是最大的，近心為次大．中央部位可觀察到Mamelon有3到5束較為細小的構造．而從切緣來看近遠心隅角部透明區域，遠心範圍較近心來得大．鄰接面方

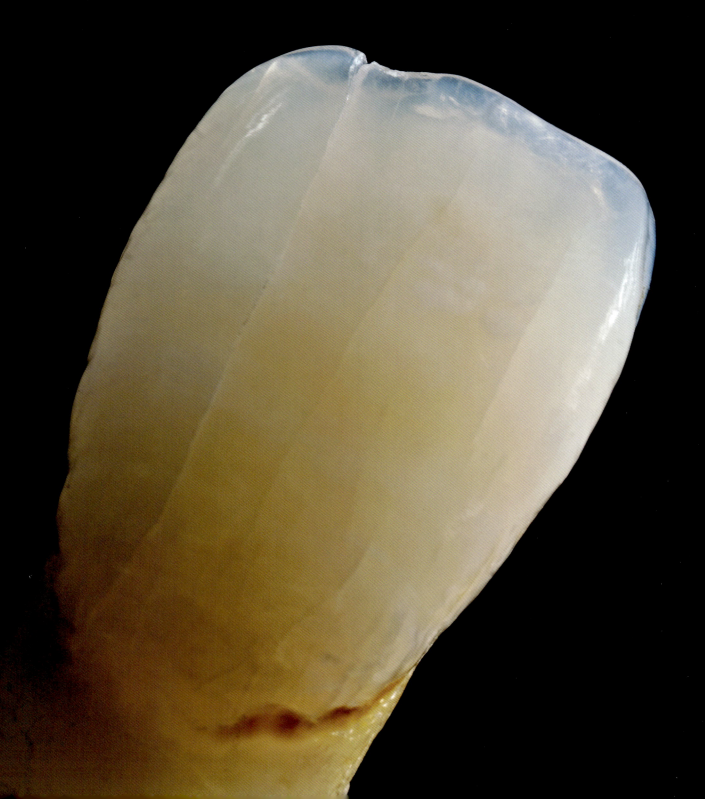

部の透明なエリアは近心に比べて遠心のほうが幅が広いものの切縁部のみに見られ，隣接面では近遠心とも強い透明性を感じない．
筆者がこのタイプの歯を表現する場合，マメロンの谷間はマメロンタイプよりも浅く表現している．またマメロン部のバックにはやや青みのある，オパール効果のある陶材でマメロン部の縁端を囲んでいる．

between these Mameron, three to five narrow Mamelon were observed. Translucent area at the medial and distal corner around an incisal edge, distal side of that area is wider than medial side. However, that phenomenon was observed only at the incisal edge, and typically in intermediate type, high transparency area was not observed at the distal and medial of contact area.
To construct intermediate type Mamelon, the shape in between Mamelon is boiled slightly shallow, and put a bluish opal effected porcelain around and/or behind of Mamelon.

面，近遠心都沒有強烈透明性．以上為此類型的特徵．
筆者在表現這類型時，在Mamelon谷間呈現上會較Mamelon型來得淺．並且Mamelon背部會稍微使用青色opal效果來圍繞切端緣．

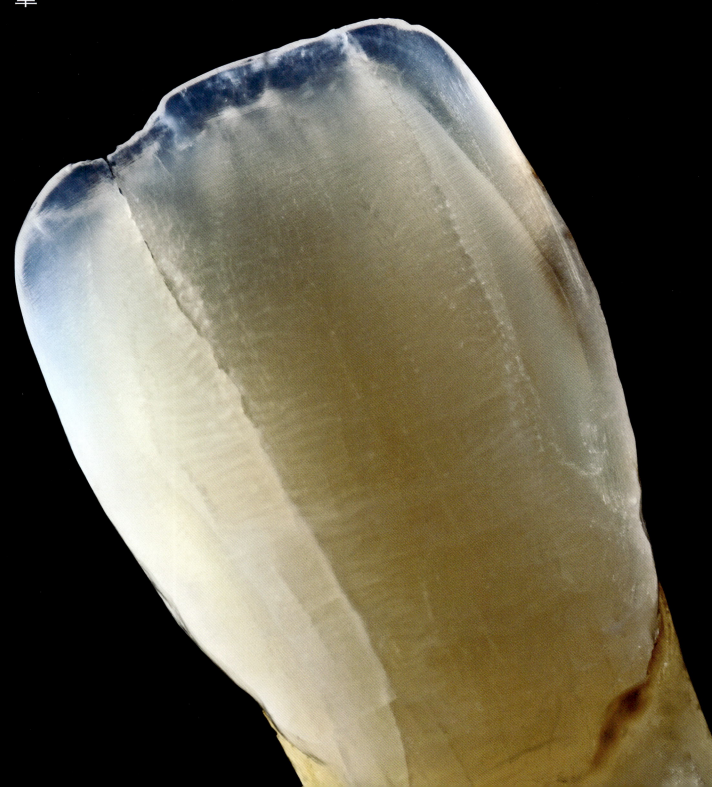

Part 3-3
Box Type

ボックスタイプの歯の特徴として，象牙質の形は歯冠形態の縮小型であることが観察できる．中央部のマメロンは観察できるが近遠心には著明なマメロンは観察されず，非常に細い縦状の構造が切縁の中央に向かって観察できる．また近遠心の隅角部の透明なエリアはほぼ同じ幅である．このタイプの歯の唇面の形態は，切縁から歯頸部にかけて彎曲が強い場合が多い．

Typical characteristic of box type shows similar shape between dentin and crown form.
The center of Mamelon is observed easily, significant shape of Mamelon is not found at medial and distal side, but very narrow shaped Mamelon is observed vertically at the center. The width of trancepearent area around the incisal corner is almost similar in between distal and medial. Furthermore in this type of tooth shows very strong corvage from incisal edge to cervical in labial side.

Box型天然牙的特徵，是象牙質的型態為牙冠型態的縮小型．中央部位可看到Mamelon，不過近遠心並不顯著，並且有非常細的縱狀構造在切緣中間呈現．近遠心透明區域幾乎相同大小．另外，此類型天然牙的唇側型態，有較多呈現切緣強烈彎曲彎向齒頸部．

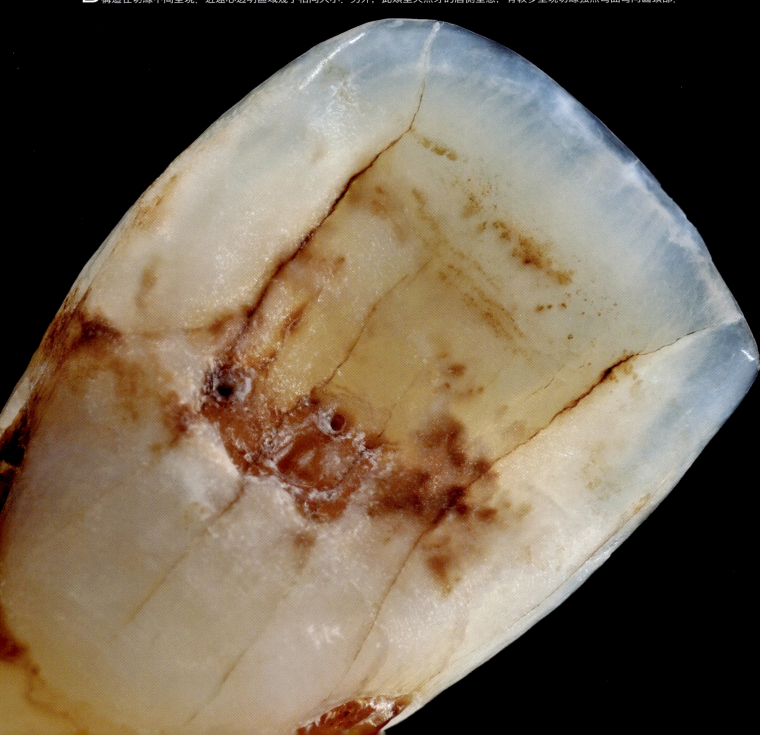

筆者がボックスタイプの歯を表現する場合，蛍光性を持たないカーキーもしくはオリーブグリーンのマメロンベースの上に，やや蛍光性のある陶材とデンティン色を混合して内部構造を表している．切縁部には乳濁色のオパール陶材を使用している．

To construct the box type, mixture porcelain of dentin color and fluorescence put over the base of Mamelon made by khaki without fluorescence or olive green porcelain.
In addition, milky opal porcelain is used at the incisal edge.

筆者在表現Box型的時候，使用不具螢光性的卡其色，或是以olive green為Mamelon base，並堆疊上略有螢光性的陶材混合著dentin一起呈現內部構造．另外，切緣部位使用乳濁色的opal陶材．

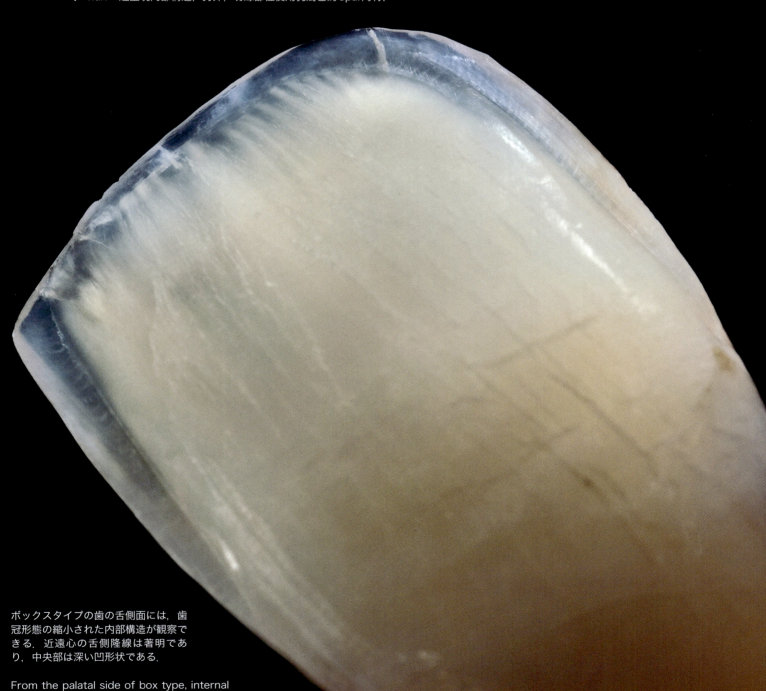

ボックスタイプの歯の舌側面には，歯冠形態の縮小された内部構造が観察できる．近遠心の舌側隆線は著明であり，中央部は深い凹形状である．

From the palatal side of box type, internal structure shows similar form as a crown contour. Medial and distal ridge is observed very clearly.

Box型天然牙的舌側內部構造是牙冠型態的縮小型．近遠心有明顯的舌側隆線，中間是較深的凹陷狀．

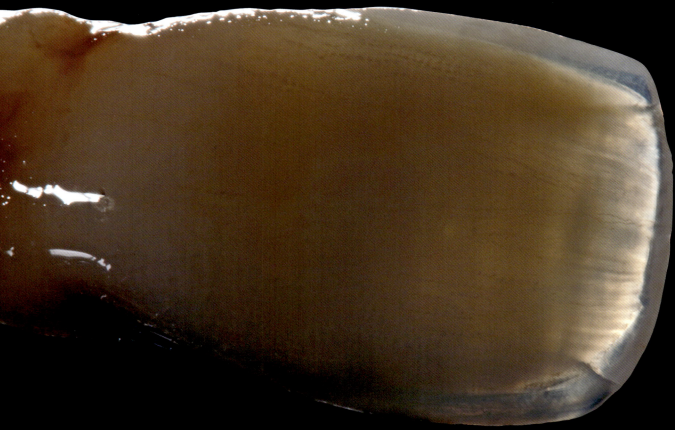

ボックスタイプの天然歯の光学特性.
非常に細かな繊維状の縦の内部構造や,エナメル質と象牙質との境界面に縦のクラックラインが多く観察できる.

The optical properties of the box type.
Small vertical fiber shaped internal structure and many vertical cracks between the enamel and dentin are observed.

Box型天然牙的光學特性.
擁有非常細小的纖維狀縱向內部構造,以及大多可觀察到琺瑯質和象牙質交界面上有縱向的 crack line.

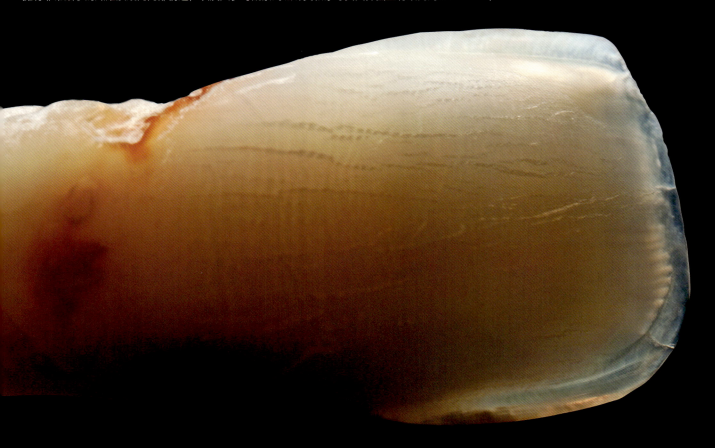

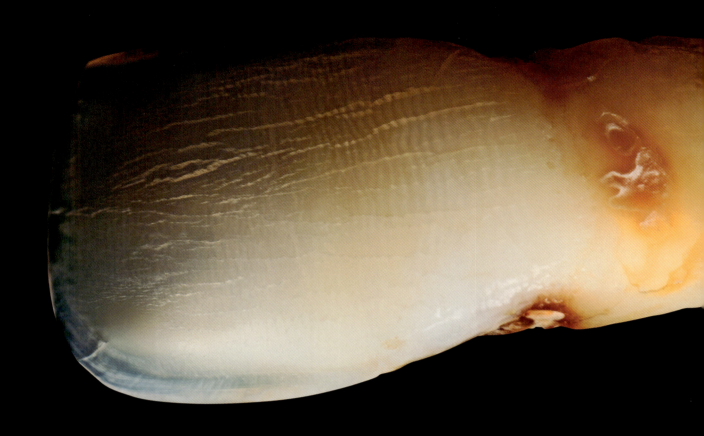
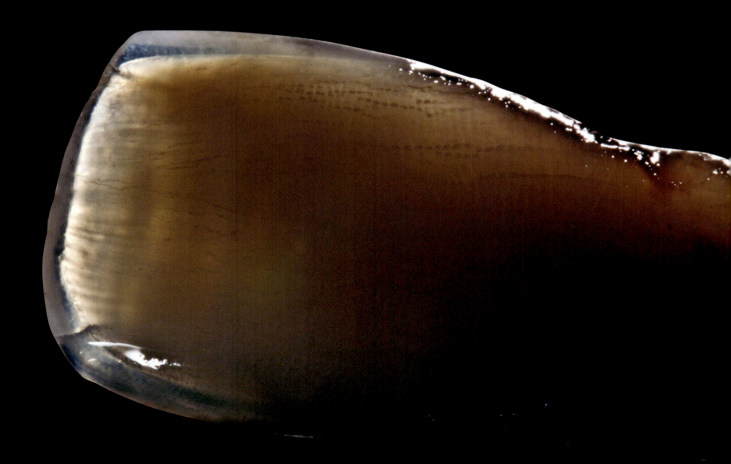

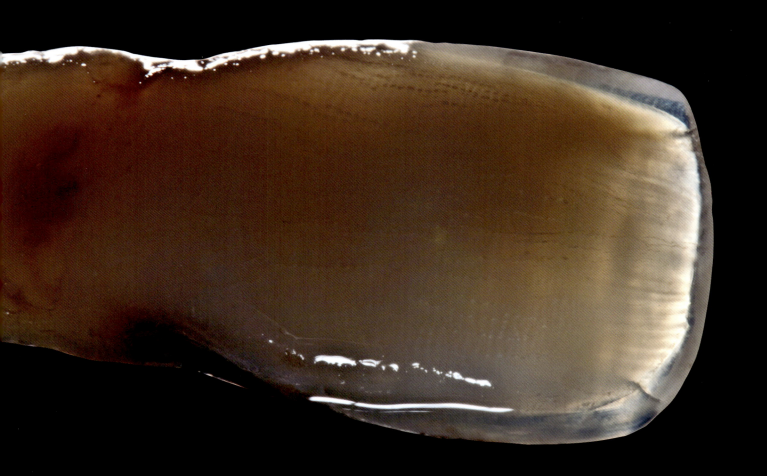
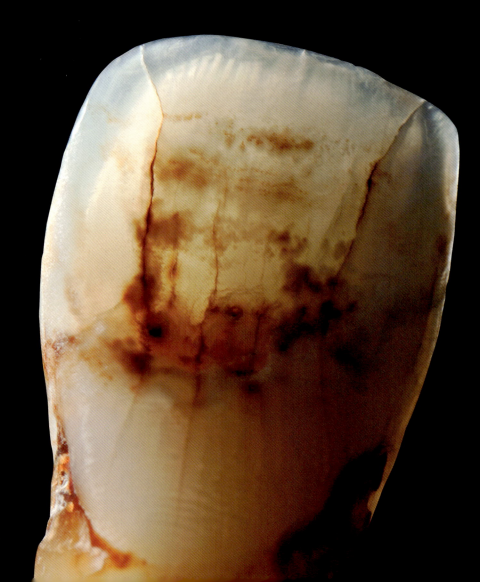

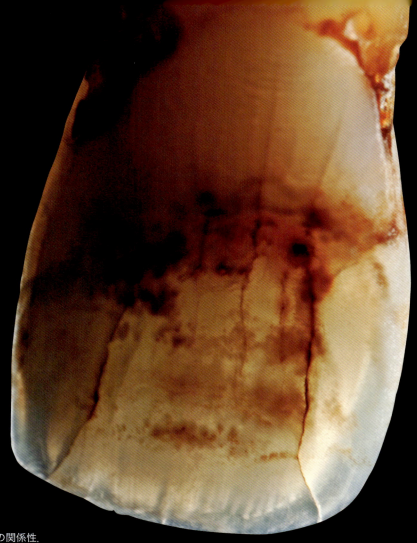

ボックスタイプの天然歯の内部構造と舌側面との関係性.

Relationship between the internal structure and the lingual surface on the box type.

Box型天然牙的內部構造與舌側關連性.

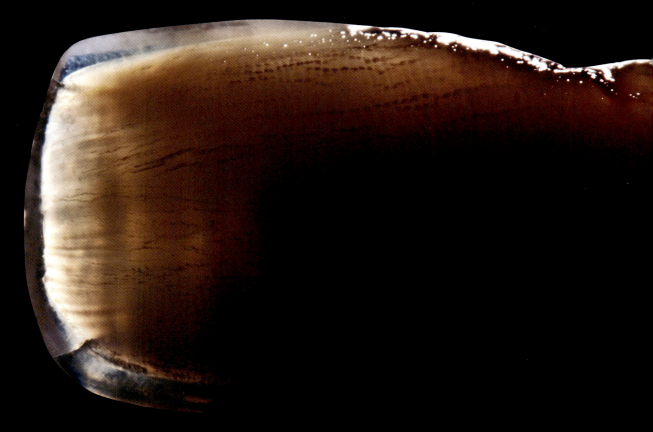

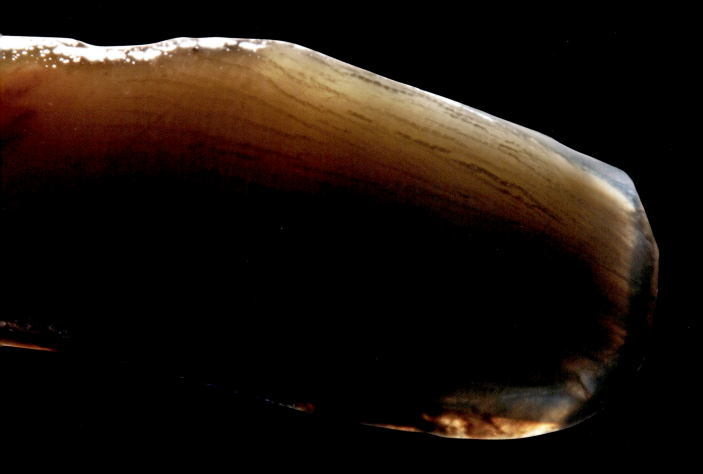

ボックスタイプの象牙質とエナメル質との境界部には縦の構造線が観察できる.
Vertical line is observed in between enamel and dentin on the box type.
Box型天然牙的象牙質和琺瑯質交界可觀察到縱向的結構線.

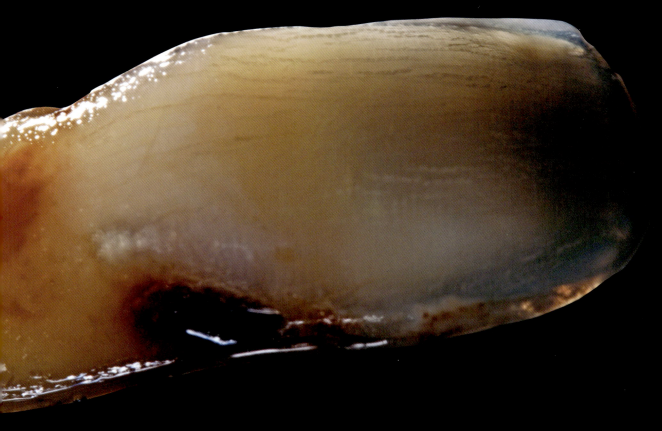

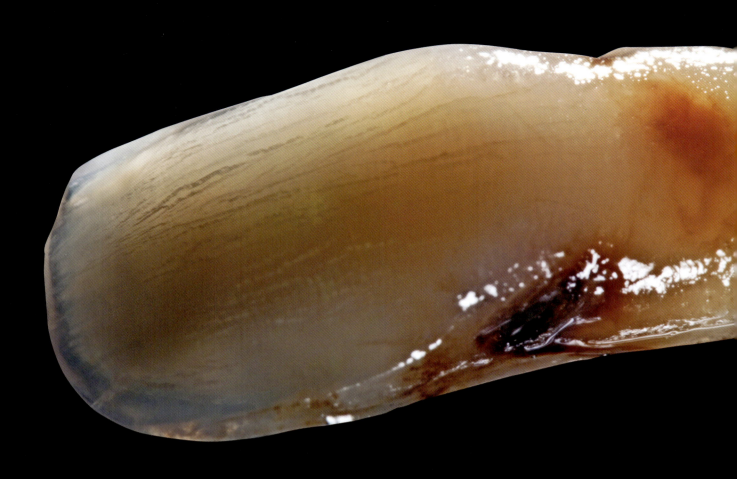
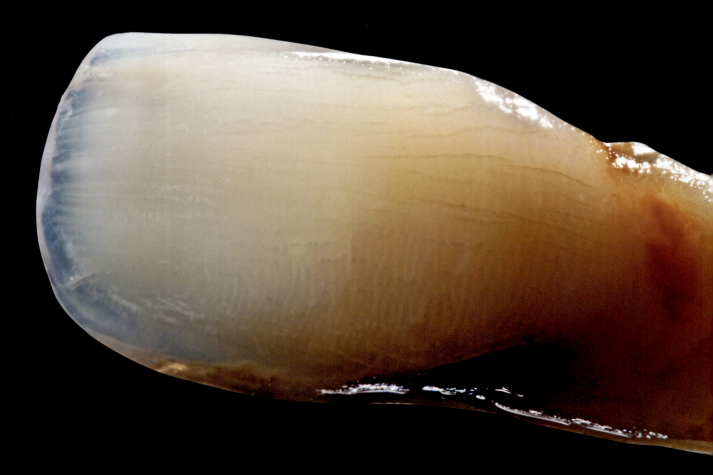

Part 3-4
Alteration

上顎前歯部の切縁が摩耗したことによる色調への影響.

The effect of wear at the incisal edge on the maxillary anterior teeth for color tone.

上顎前齒的切緣因磨耗而影響到色調.

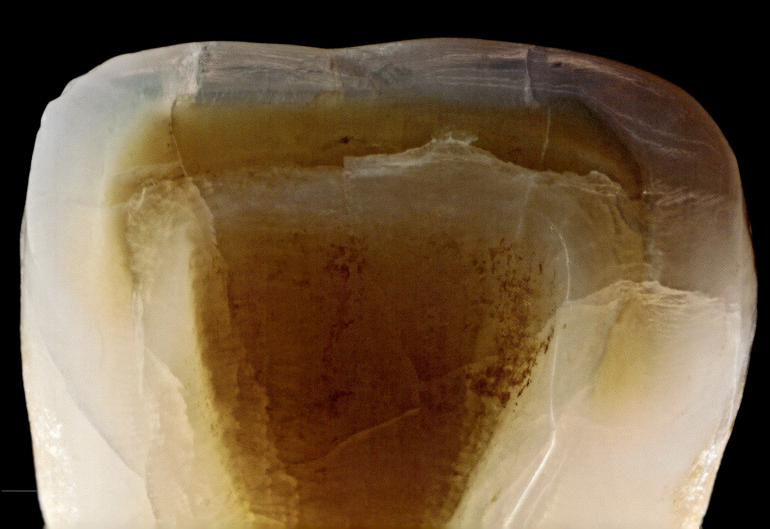

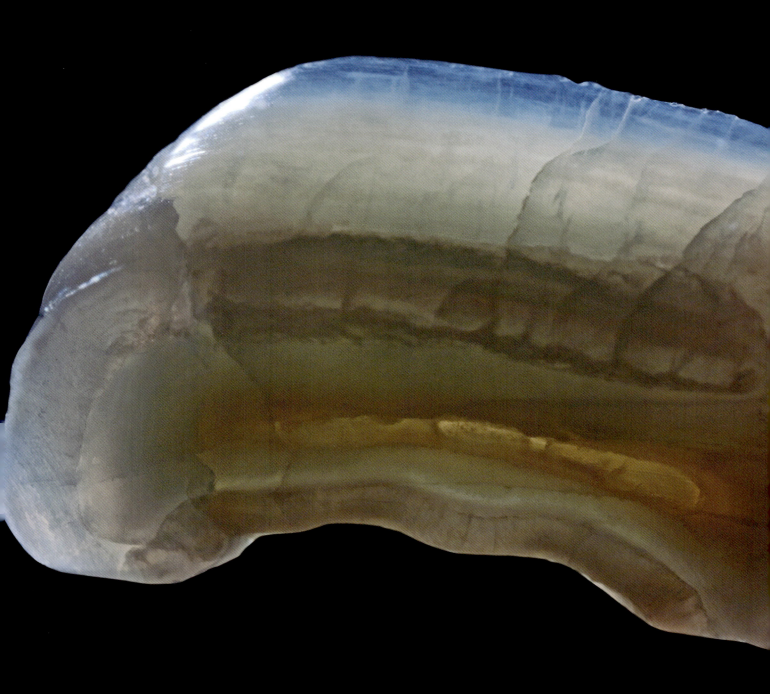

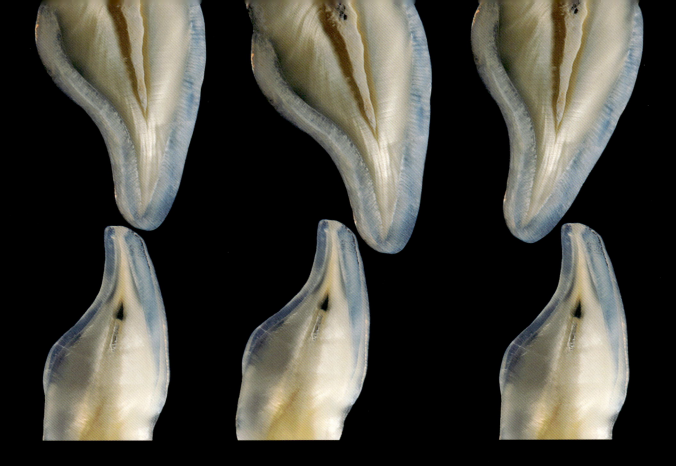

Dr.Frank Spearの前歯部の咬合関係による摩耗の分類.

Classification of occlusal wear at the anterior region by Dr.Frank Spear.

Dr.Frank Spear依前齒的咬合關係進行磨耗分類.

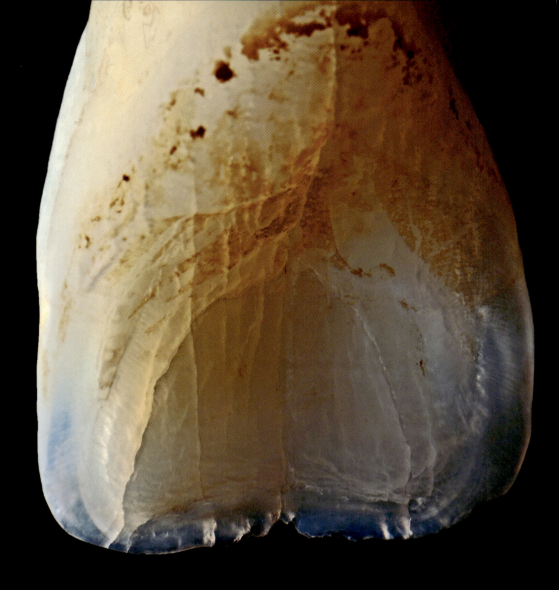
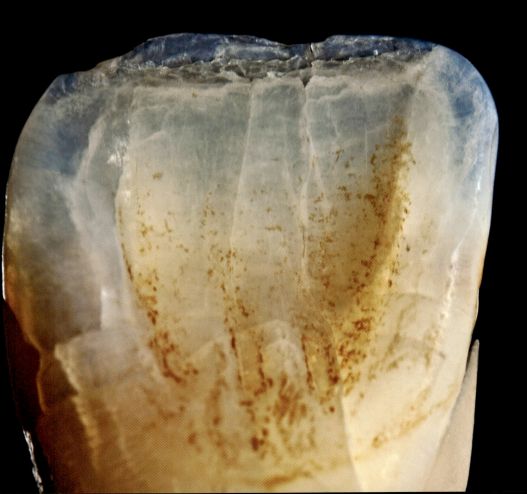

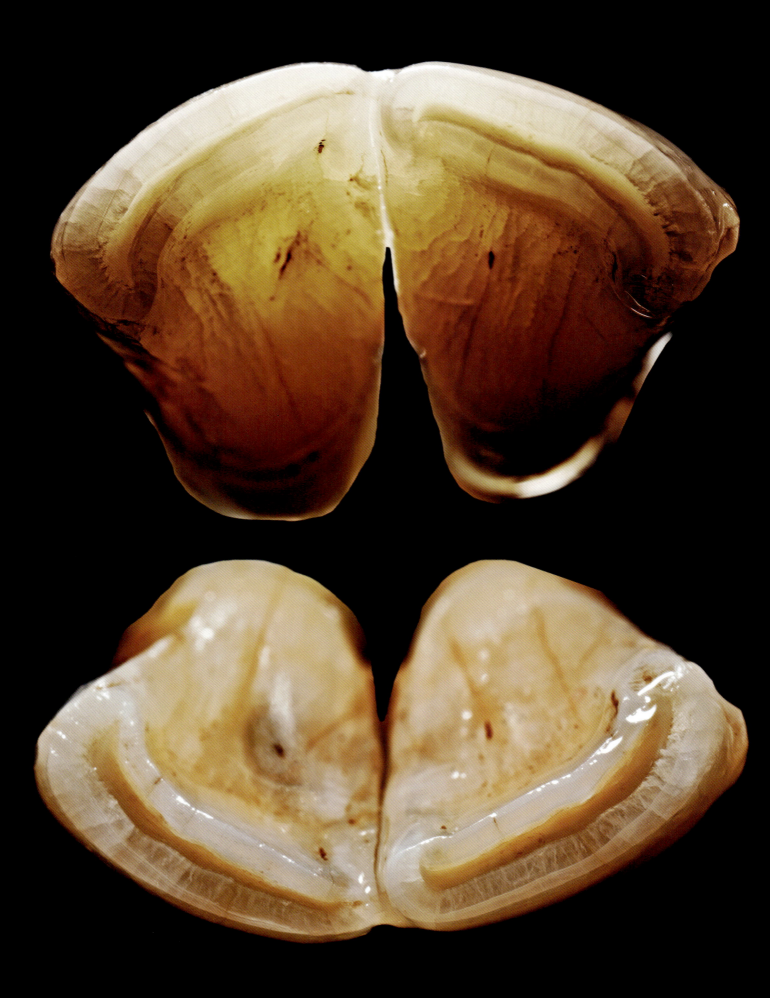

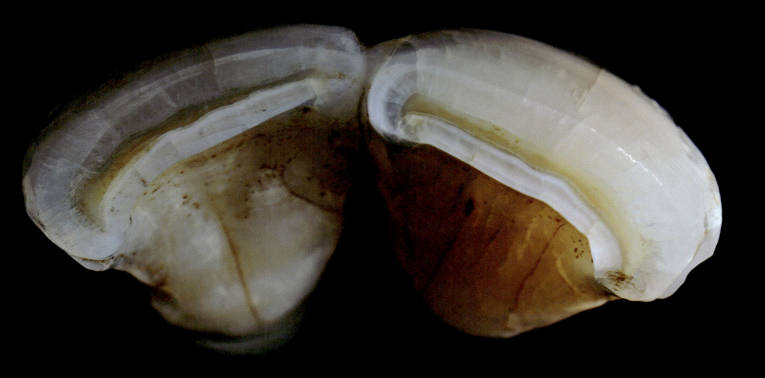

連続した上顎中切歯の切縁の摩耗.

Continuous wear at the incisal edge of maxillary central incisor.

上顎中門齒連續性切緣磨耗.

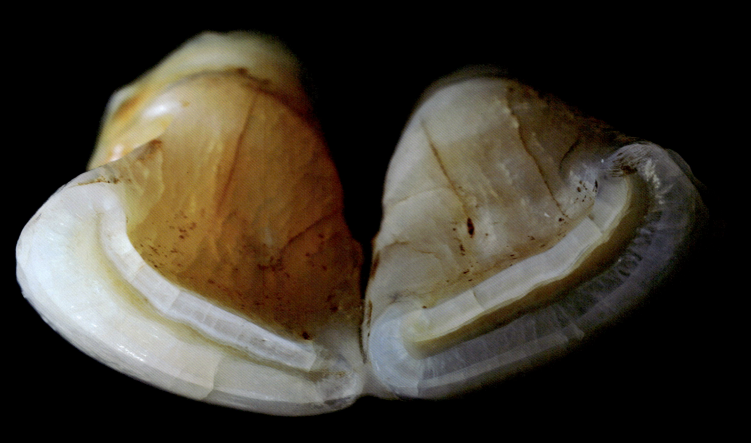

因上顎中門齒的連續性切緣磨耗所形成二次象牙質，提高了琺瑯質透明性．

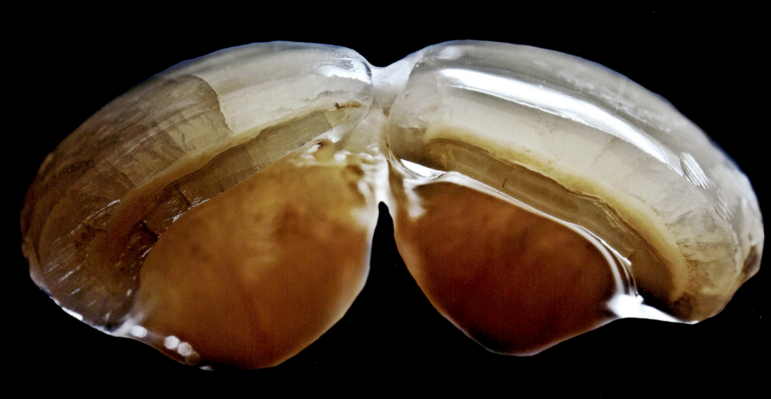

連続した上顎中切歯の切縁の摩耗により，二次象牙質が形成されることで，エナメル質の透明性が高くなっている．

The transparency of the enamel is getting higher because of secondary dentin made by continuous wear at the incisal edge of maxillary central incisor.

因上顎中門齒的連續性切緣磨耗所形成二次象牙質，提高了琺瑯質透明性．

因切縁的磨耗，可觀察到琺瑯質深入到象牙質表面的裂紋，也因此阻斷光對琺瑯質的透射．

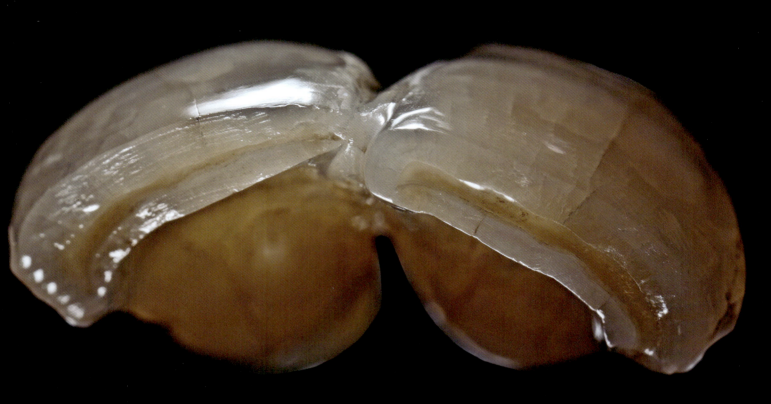

切縁の摩耗により，エナメル質も象牙質表面までの深いクラックが観察できる．また深いクラックによりエナメル質の光の透過性が遮断されていることも観察される．

The wear of the incisal edge, deep crack made by tooth wear is observed at the surface of dentin under the enamel. Also transmitted light is blocked by the deep crack is observed.

因切縁的磨耗，可觀察到琺瑯質深入到象牙質表面的裂紋，也因此阻斷光對琺瑯質的透射．

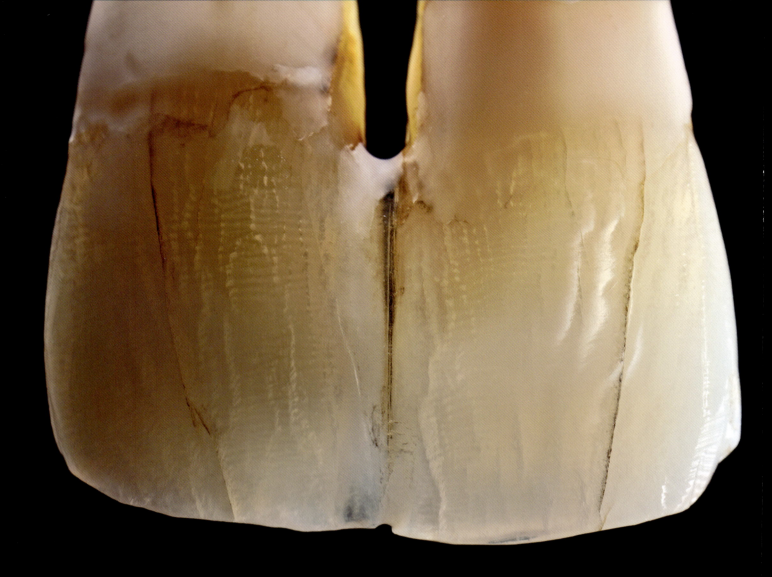
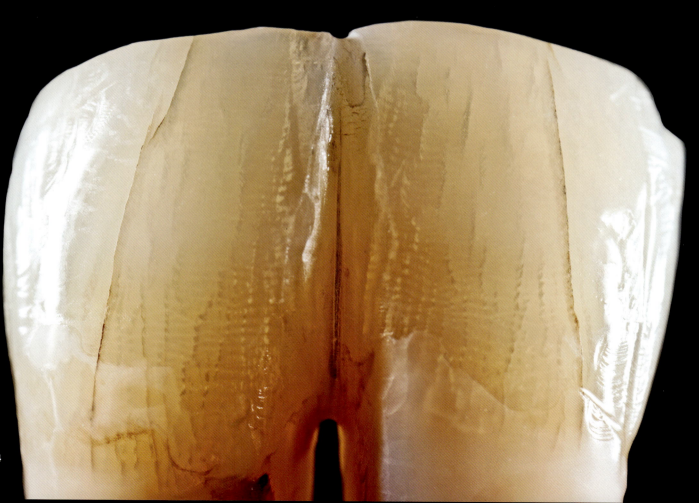

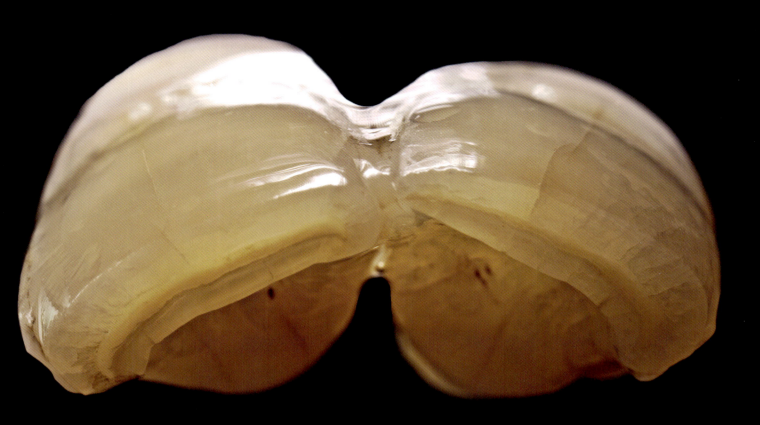

天然歯はエナメル質が摩耗することにより,象牙質及び歯髄腔が二次象牙質へと変化(ガラス化)し,歯冠の色調に変化が現れる.

The stress which forced from tooth wear, affect to the dentin and pulp to be the secondary dentin, and it will be affected tooth color change.

天然牙的琺瑯質受到磨損,使得象牙質及牙髓腔形成二次象牙質玻璃化,產生了牙冠色調上的變化.

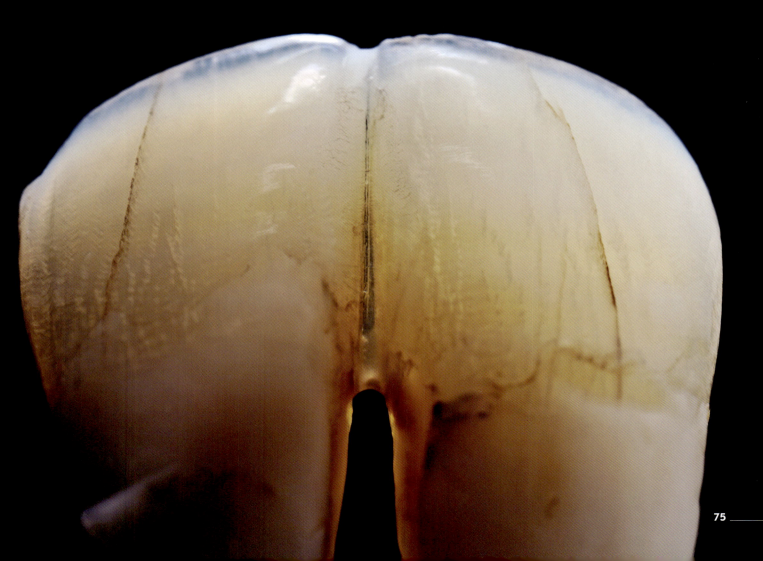

Part 3-5
Anterior Root

上顎中切歯の歯根から切縁までをスライスしてエリアごとに観察した.

Cross sectional observation of the maxillary central incisor.

上顎中門齒從牙根到切緣部進行區域性切片觀察.

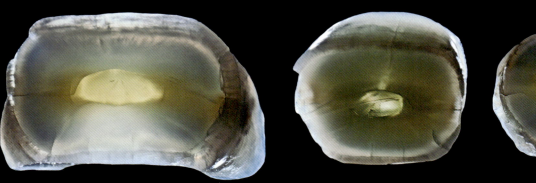
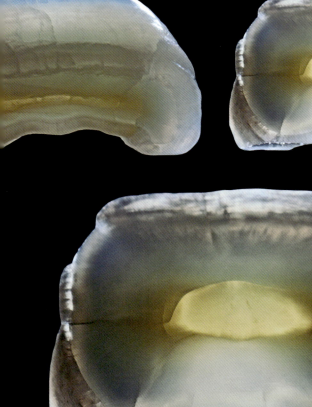

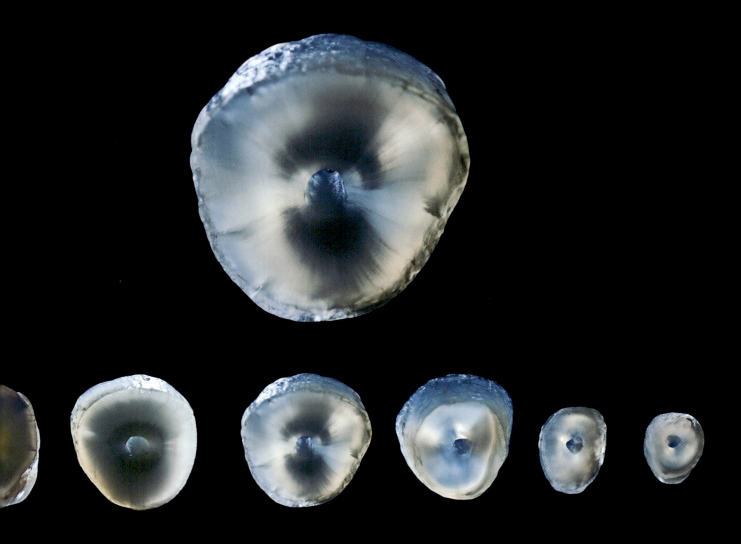

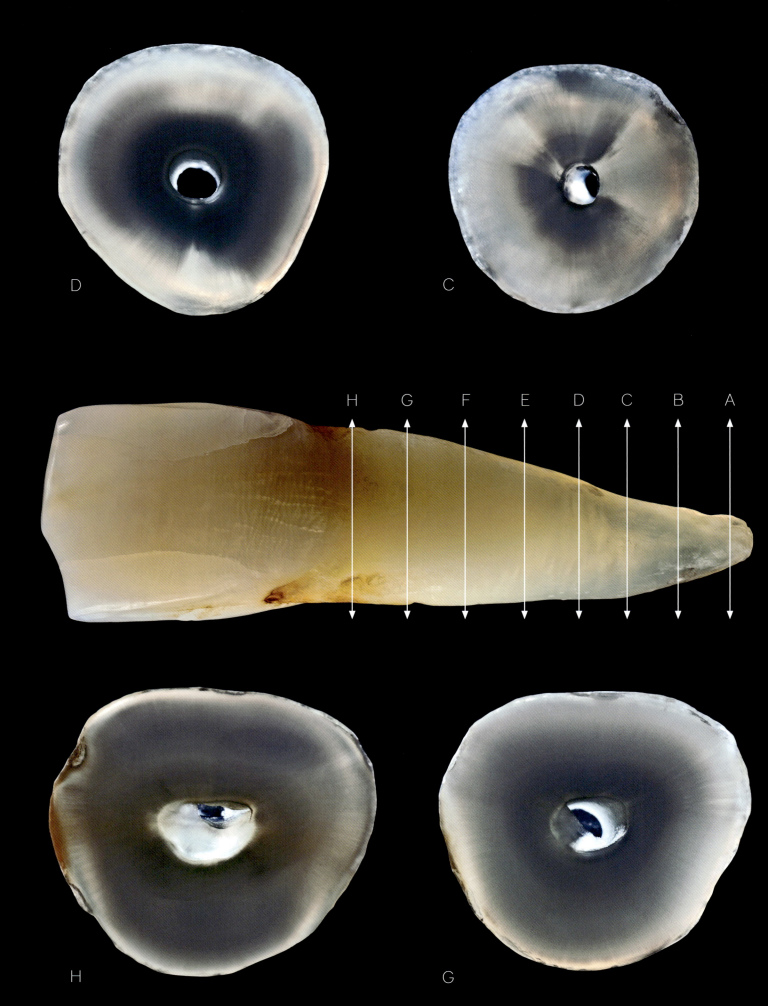

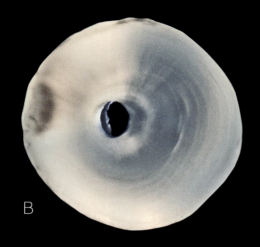
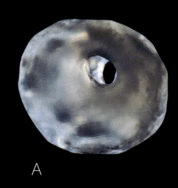

歯頸部付近までは歯髄腔が観察できる.

Pulp can be observed from root apex to cervical area.

在齒頸部附近可以觀察到牙髓腔.

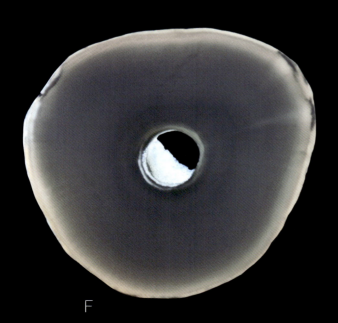
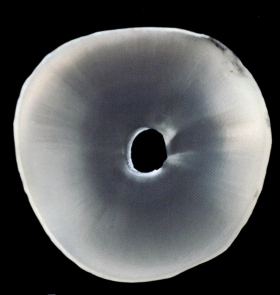

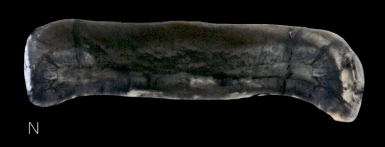

N

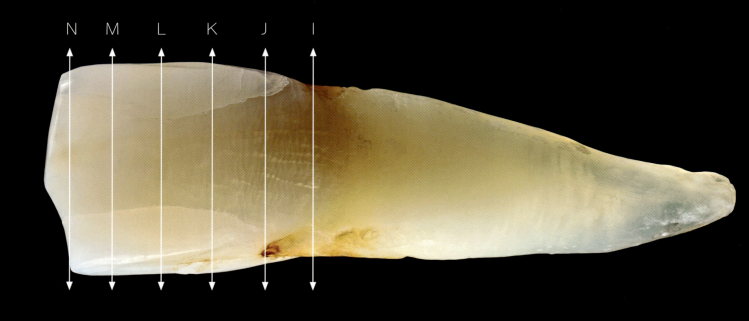

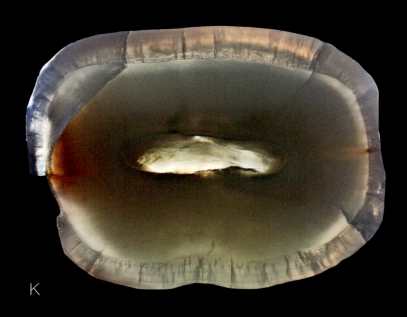

K

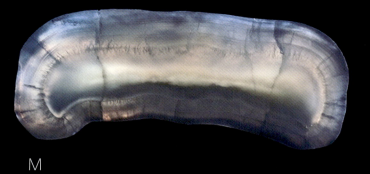 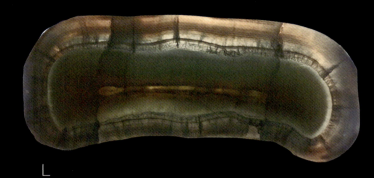

この歯の歯頸部から切縁までは歯髄腔が石灰化しているのが観察できる．

The pulp which calcified from cervical to incisal edge is observed.

從齒頸部到切緣，可觀察到牙髓腔鈣化現象．

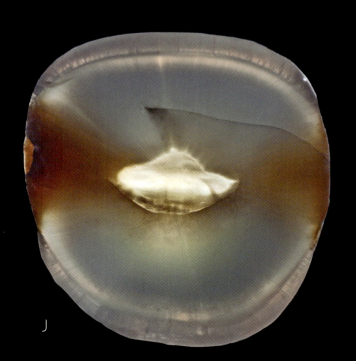 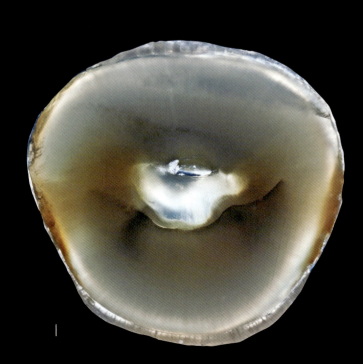

二次象牙質

Secondary dentin

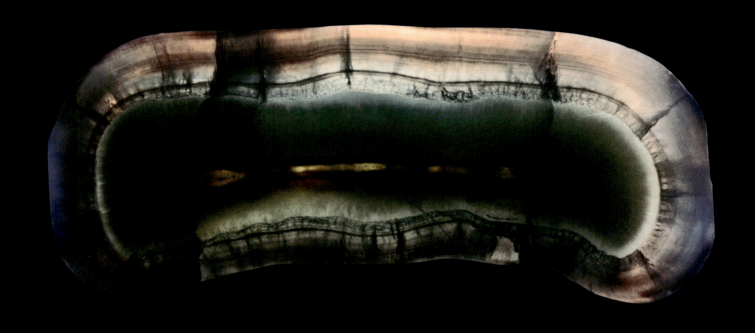

二次象牙質

Secondary dentin

二次象牙質

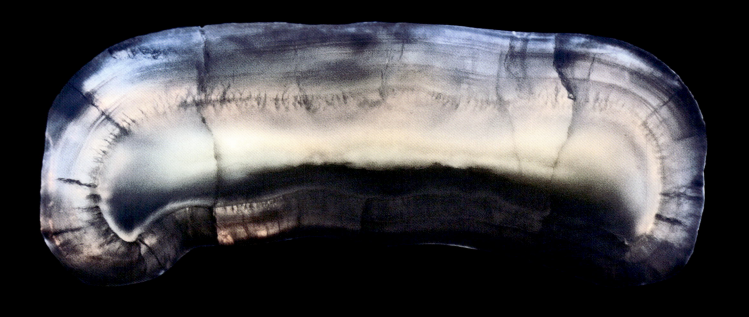

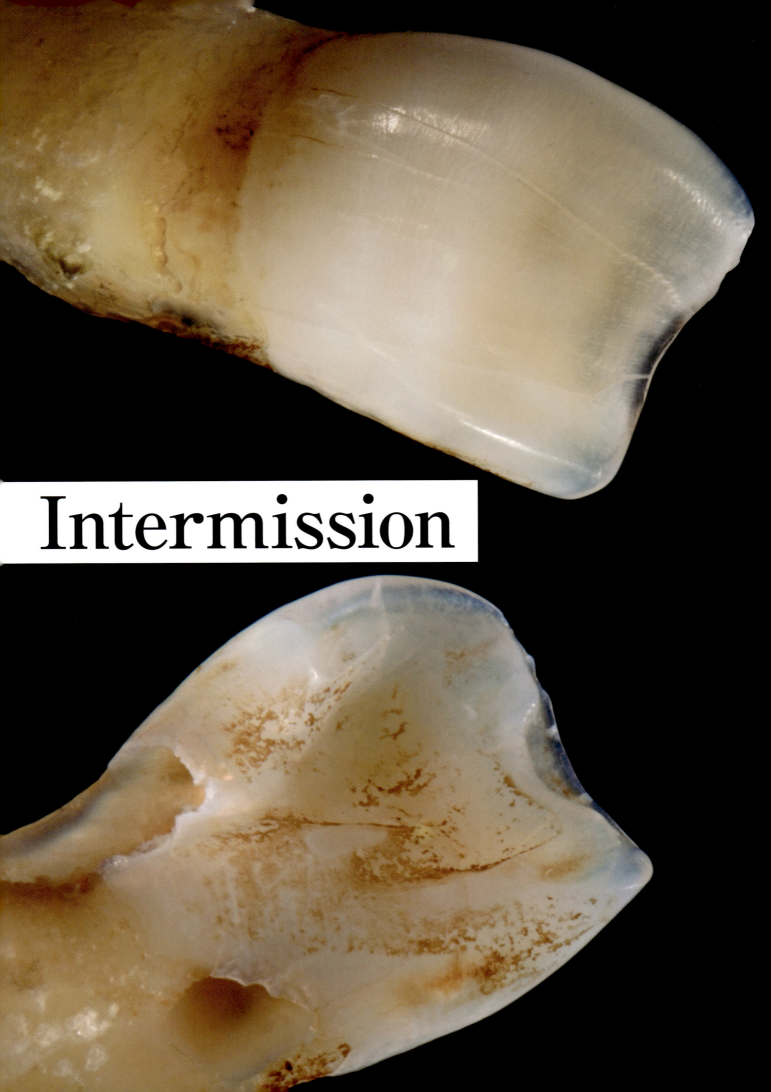

Intermission

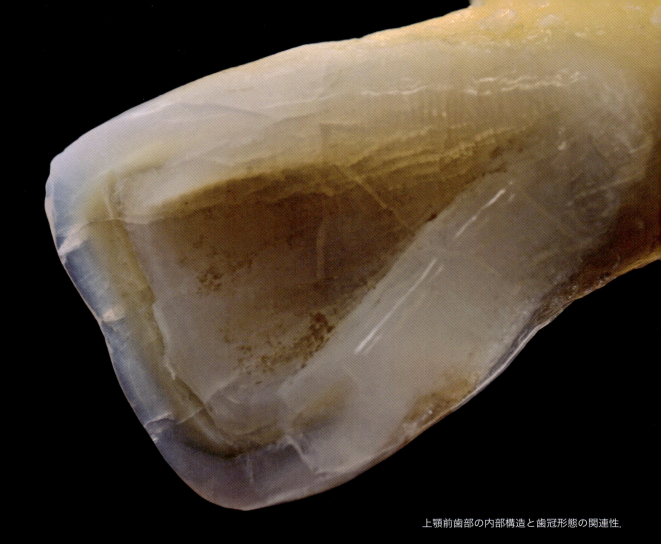

上顎前歯部の内部構造と歯冠形態の関連性.
The relationship between tooth morphology and internal structure in maxillary anterior teeth.
上顎前齒內部構造與牙冠型態的關係.

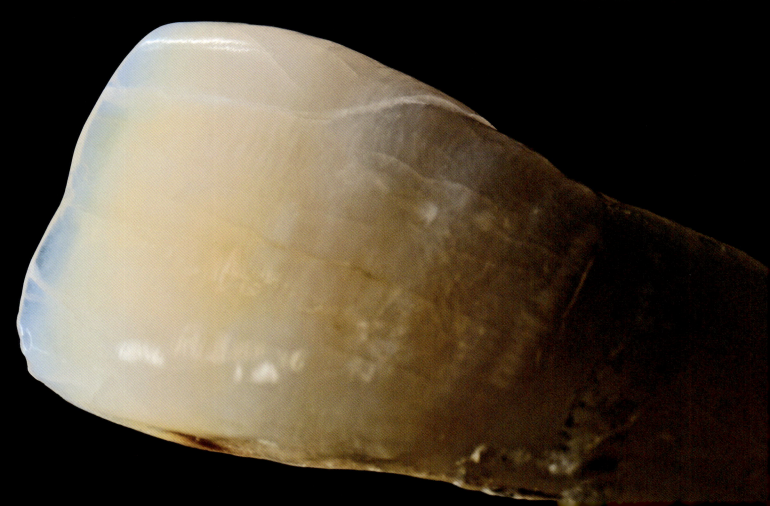

Part 4-1
Devil Head M Type

デビルヘッドタイプの歯の特徴として，切縁のファセットにより，象牙質が石灰化して歯冠の透明性が高くなっている．特に切縁から歯冠中央部では象牙質の明度が低下しているのが理解できる．内部構造は，縦状のものよりも近遠心にかけての三日月状あるいは半月状の，灰色の象牙質が観察できる．これはマメロンタイプの歯が経年的に変化することで見られる特徴であるので，基本的にはマメロンタイプのそれを"継承"しているが，歯冠内部のガラス化も進んでいることから，歯冠全体の明度は低下している．

The characteristics of Devil head type show high transparency because tooth wear at the edge affected to pulp modified as a calcificated dentin, and lower brightness of dentin is observed especially around edge to center of crown. Internal structure of Devil head type, grayish half-moon-shaped dentin can be observed easily around medial and distal area. Devil head type is also categorized as a group of Mameron type, so it shows typical characteristics of Mameron type. Overall, the color of crown shows lower brightness because an internal structure of crown is changed as glassy color.

Devil Head型的特徵是，由於切緣的facet，可觀察到象牙質的鈣化現象提高了牙冠的透明度．特別是可以了解到，切緣到牙冠中央部位的象牙質明度是下降的．近遠心的內部構造可觀察到新月狀或半月狀的灰色的象牙質色調。經由Mamelon型所變化而來，因此繼承了Mamelon型的特徵，也可觀察到牙冠內部的玻璃化使得牙冠整體明度下降．

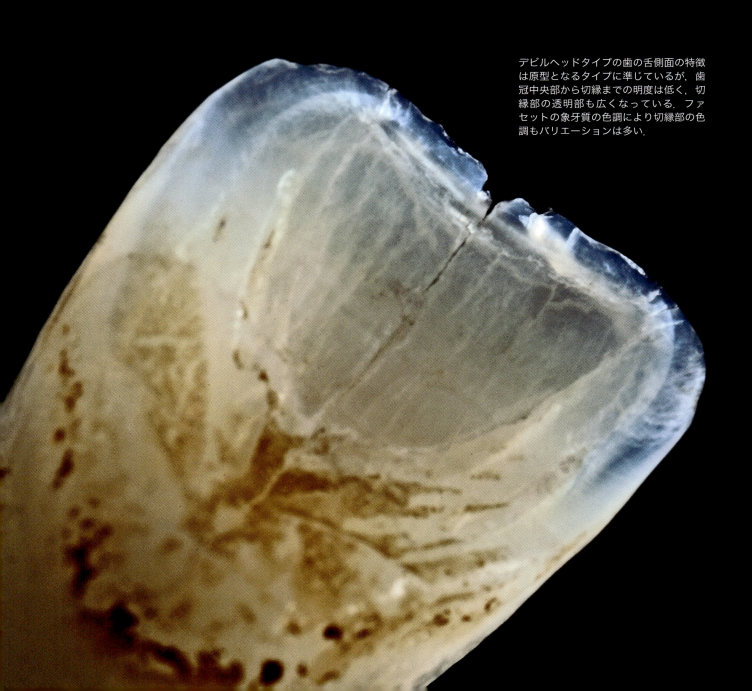

デビルヘッドタイプの歯の舌側面の特徴は原型となるタイプに準じているが，歯冠中央部から切縁までの明度は低く，切縁部の透明部も広くなっている．ファセットの象牙質の色調により切縁部の色調もバリエーションは多い．

デビルヘッドタイプの表現は簡単ではないと言えよう．サンプルでの製作はできるのだが，口腔内の隣在歯と調和したキャラクター及び明度，彩度までを近似させるのは，直接シェードテイキングを行うか質の高い口腔内写真が必要となる．このようなことからも，筆者はこの歯のタイプに「デビル」との呼称を与えた次第である．

To create characteristics of Devil head type for prosthetic is not easy. It is possible to construct "similar" characteristics, but to perform the perfect match as a natural teeth which shows a harmony of brightness and chroma, carful char-side observation and/or perfect picture with some different angles are recommended. It was named as the Devil head also from such a reason.

技術上要表現Devil Head型並不容易．也許可以模仿樣本進行製作，不過為了與口腔內鄰牙的特徵或明度彩度作調和，必需直接進行shade taking並拍攝畫質好的照片．也因製作上困難而有惡魔之稱號．

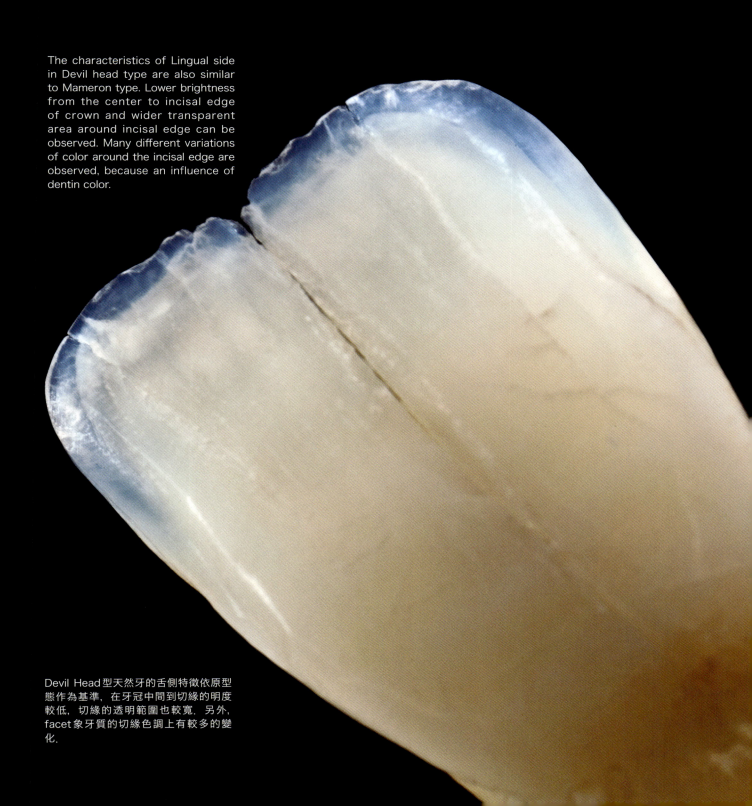

The characteristics of Lingual side in Devil head type are also similar to Mameron type. Lower brightness from the center to incisal edge of crown and wider transparent area around incisal edge can be observed. Many different variations of color around the incisal edge are observed, because an influence of dentin color.

Devil Head型天然牙的舌側特徵依原型態作為基準，在牙冠中間到切緣的明度較低，切緣的透明範圍也較寬．另外，facet象牙質的切緣色調上有較多的變化．

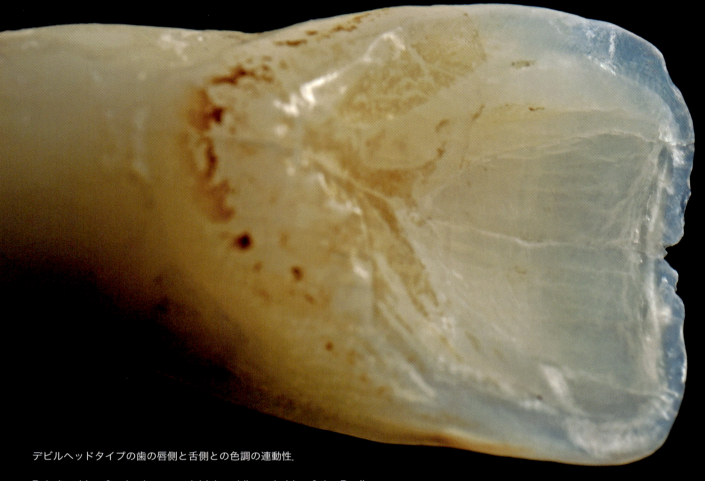

デビルヘッドタイプの歯の唇側と舌側との色調の連動性.

Relationship of color between labial and lingual side of the Devil head type.

Devil Head型天然牙的唇側與舌側色調上的關連性.

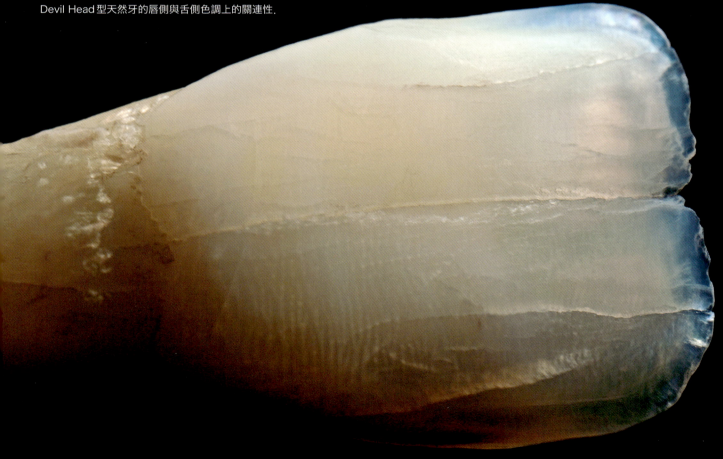

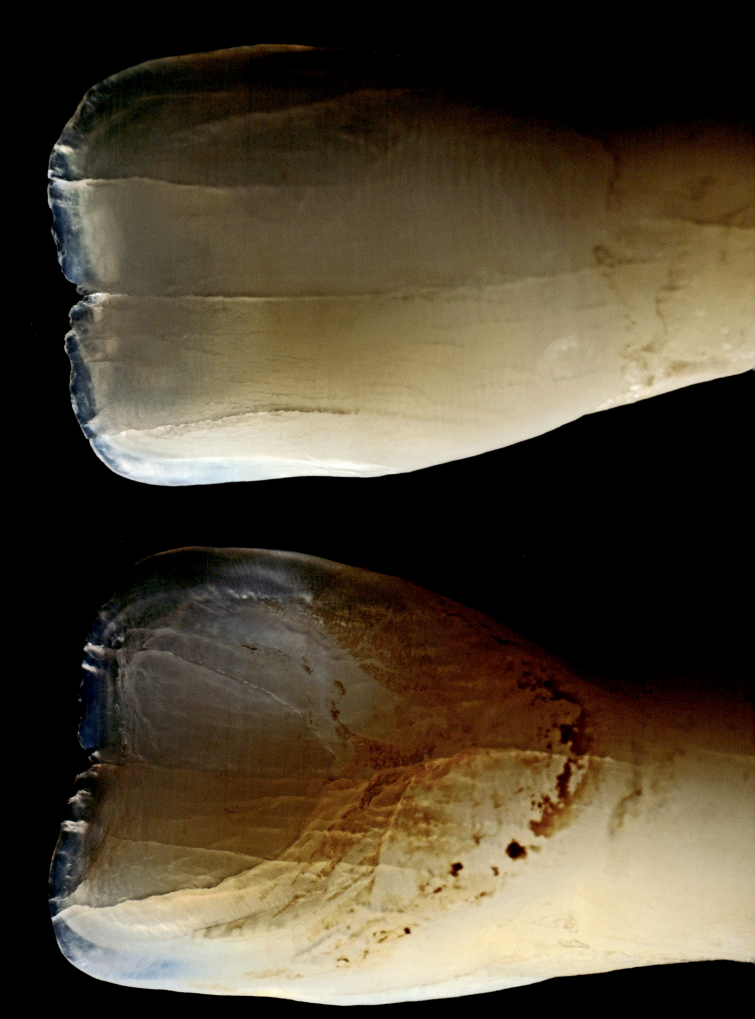

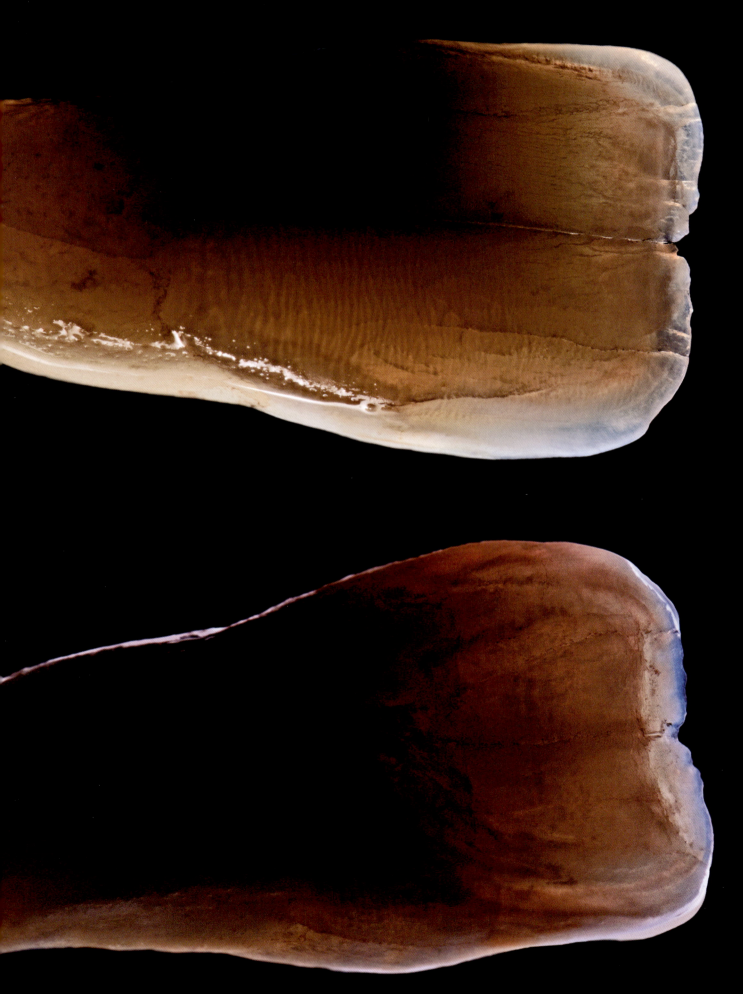

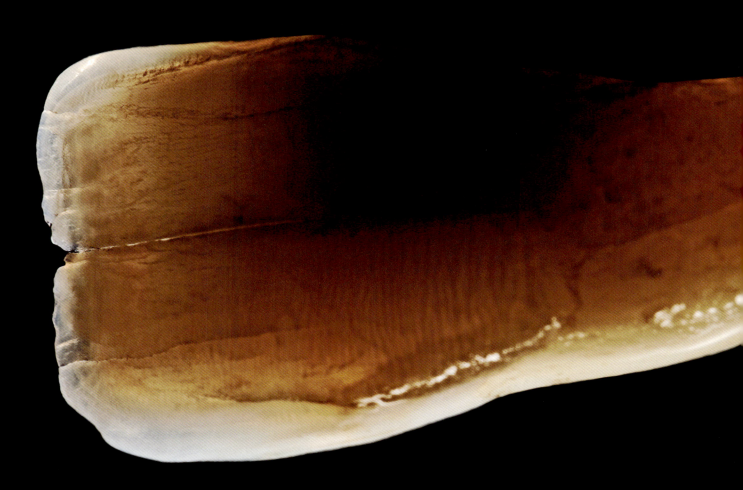

デビルヘッドタイプでは象牙質表面と残存エナメル質のオパール効果が高まっている．

The Devil head type shows strong opal effect at the enamel and dentin surface.

Devil Head型的象牙質表面和殘存琺瑯質有較高的opal效果．

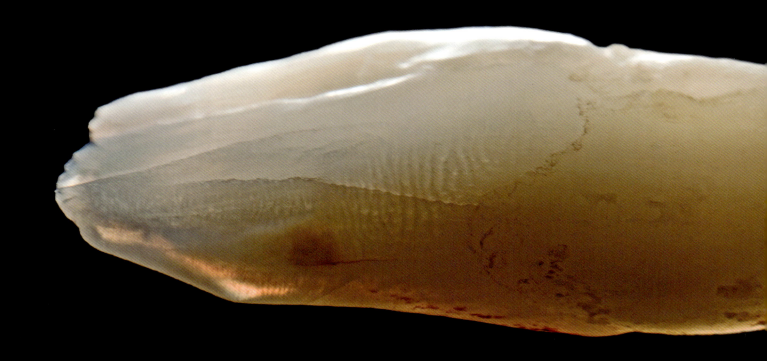

Part 4-2
Devil Head B Type

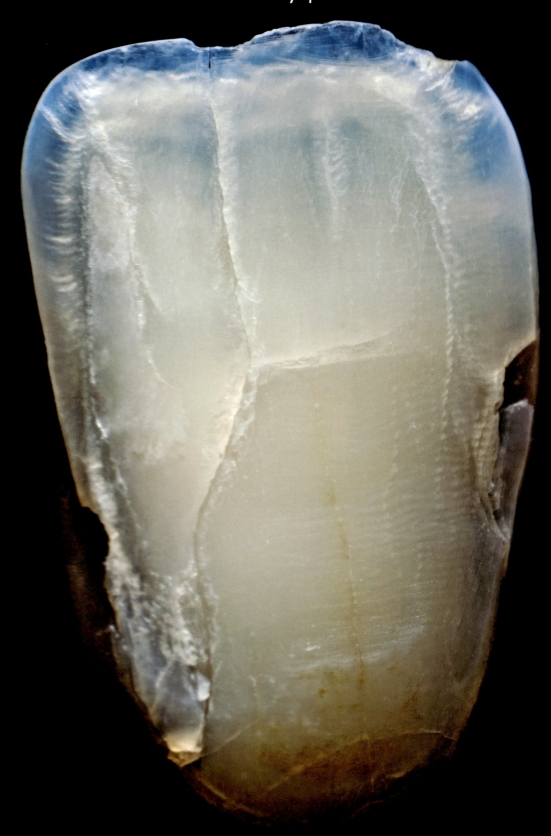

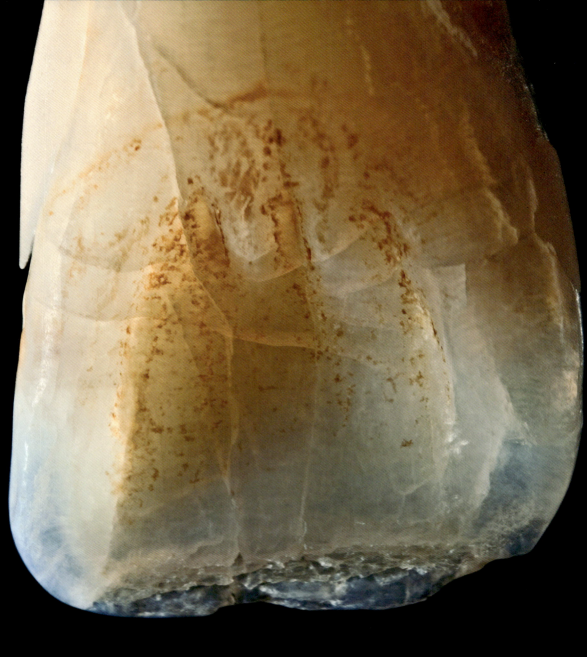

デビルヘッドBタイプの歯の特徴として，ボックスタイプの歯の特徴を継承している．切縁のファセットにより，象牙質の石灰化に伴う歯冠の透明性の変化については，マメロンタイプよりもやや少なく感じる．しかしながら，切縁〜歯冠中央部の明度は低くなり，透明性はやや高くなっている．デビルヘッドBタイプの最大の特徴として，歯冠中央部から歯頸部の明度の低下が観察されにくいことが挙げられる．おそらく，ボックスタイプの特徴的な歯冠形態もこの色調の変化に関与していると考えられる．

The characteristics of Devil head B type show high transparency because tooth wear at the edge affected to pulp modified as a calcificated dentin, and lower brightness of dentin is observed especially around edge to center of crown. Devil Head Type B shows similar characteristics as Box type, and transparency change is smaller than the Mameron type. However lower brightness and higher transparency is observed from incisal edge to center of crown. Main characteristics of Devil head B type shows lower brightness change from the center of crown to the cervical area. Typically, crown shape of box type might be related with this color change.

Devil HeadB型天然牙的特徵承續著Box型的特徵，也因為切緣的facet造成象牙質鈣化現象，使得牙冠透明感略接近於Mamelon型，因此切緣到牙冠中央的明度低，透明度略偏高．Devil HeadB型最大特徵應是難以觀察到牙冠中央到齒頸部的明度下降，也許這種色調上的變化與Box型的牙冠型態有所關連．

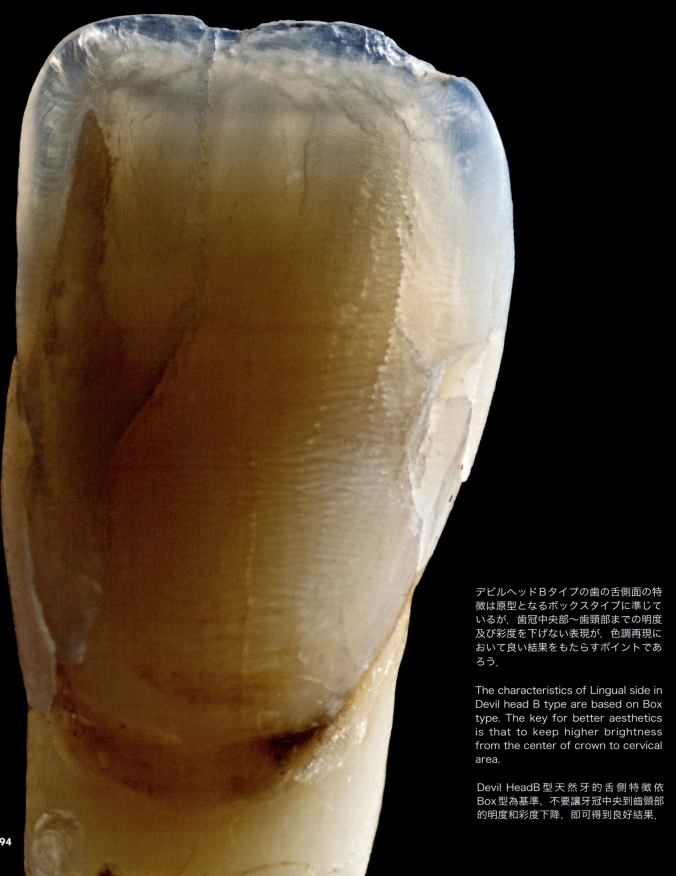

デビルヘッドBタイプの歯の舌側面の特徴は原型となるボックスタイプに準じているが，歯冠中央部〜歯頸部までの明度及び彩度を下げない表現が，色調再現において良い結果をもたらすポイントであろう．

The characteristics of Lingual side in Devil head B type are based on Box type. The key for better aesthetics is that to keep higher brightness from the center of crown to cervical area.

Devil HeadB型天然牙的舌側特徵依Box型為基準，不要讓牙冠中央到齒頸部的明度和彩度下降，即可得到良好結果．

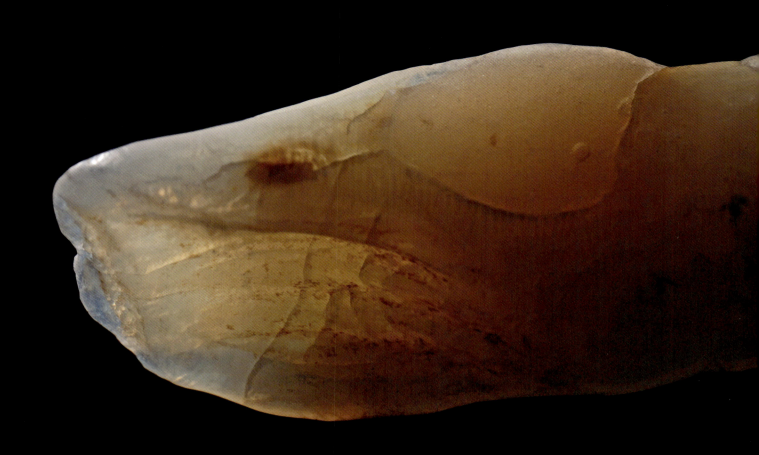
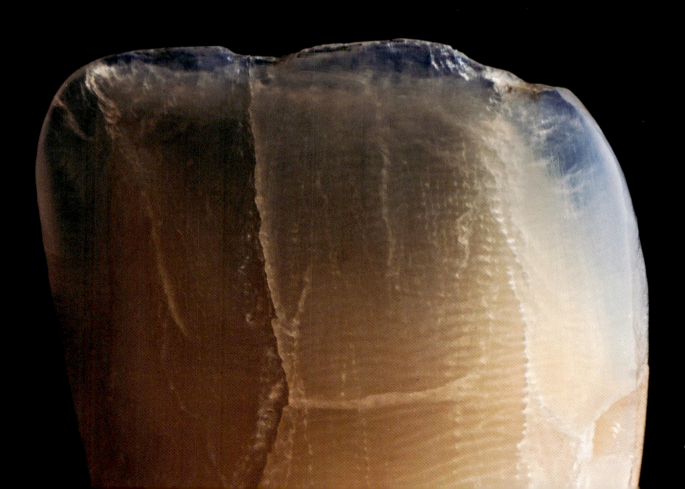

デビルヘッドBタイプの表現では，歯頸部〜歯冠中央部までの色調再現はマメロンやボックスタイプと同様な表現として，歯冠中央部〜切縁までの彩度及び明度を下げた表現が適当だと筆者は考えている．すなわち，内部構造の近心〜遠心の隅角までを，低明度で蛍光性を持たない陶材によって半月状に表現している．

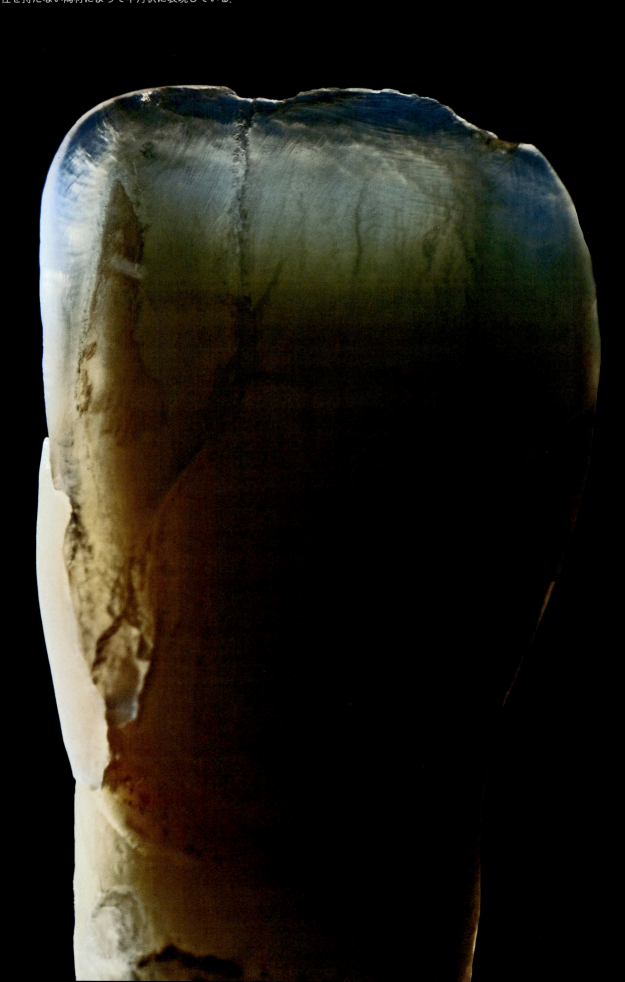

デビルヘッドBタイプの表現では，歯頸部〜歯冠中央部までの色調再現はマメロンやボックスタイプと同様な表現として，歯冠中央部〜切縁までの彩度及び明度を下げた表現が適当だと筆者は考えている．すなわち，内部構造の近心〜遠心の隅角までを，低明度で蛍光性を持たない陶材によって半月状に表現している．

Color reproduction around cervical and center of crown in Devil head B type is similar as Mameron and/or Box type. From the center of crown to incisal edge, it should be better to create as high chroma with low brightness. Internal structure from medial to distal area, porcelain without brightness and fluorescent is used as half-moon-shape.

Devil HeadB型色調的呈現，從齒頸部到牙冠中央相同於Mamelon或是Box型，牙冠中央到切緣有其彩度且明度低的方式呈現．內部構造方面，近心到遠心的隅角使用無明度無螢光性的陶材做半月狀呈現．

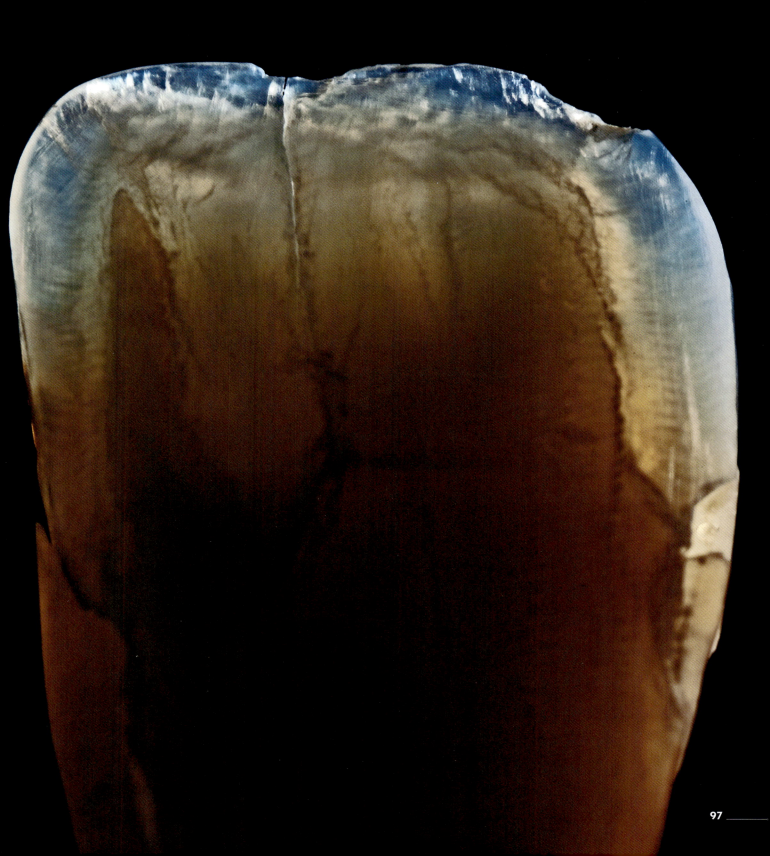

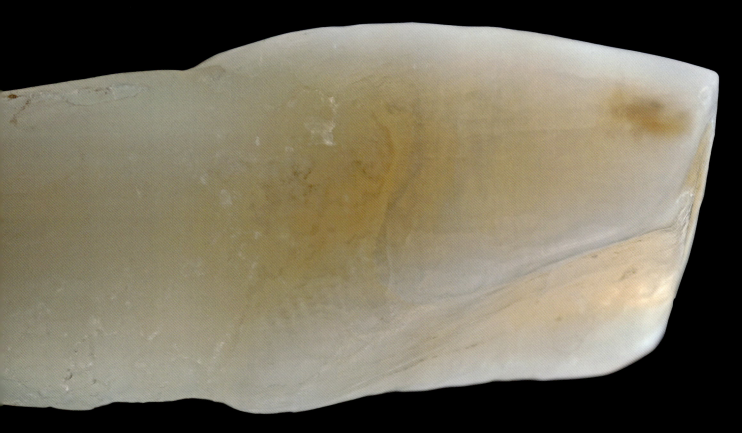

Part 5
Taper Type

テーパータイプとは，切縁の歯冠幅に対して歯頸部の幅が著しく狭くなる形態を取る，上顎前歯の形態である．もちろん，摩耗する前の歯の切縁の形状は様々であろうが，摩耗により歯のテーパー形状が特に感じられる．よってこのタイプは後天的な派生タイプであると考えられる．

Taper type is the shape of maxillary anterior teeth which has very narrow cervical width compare to the width of incisal edge. Although there are many different shape of incisal edge, tapered shape is emphasized by tooth wear. Therefore this type is acquired derivation type.

Taper 型上顎前牙的齒頸部寬度相對於切緣寬度狹小許多．當然在磨耗前切緣有種種形狀，磨耗之後更顯現其錐狀，因此這類型屬於後天性的．

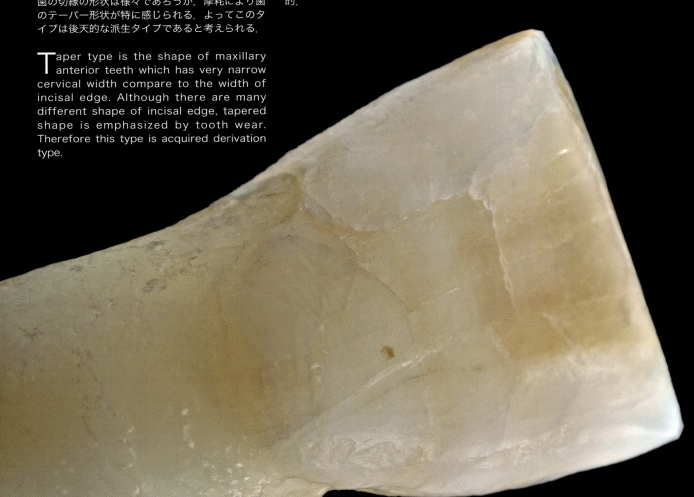

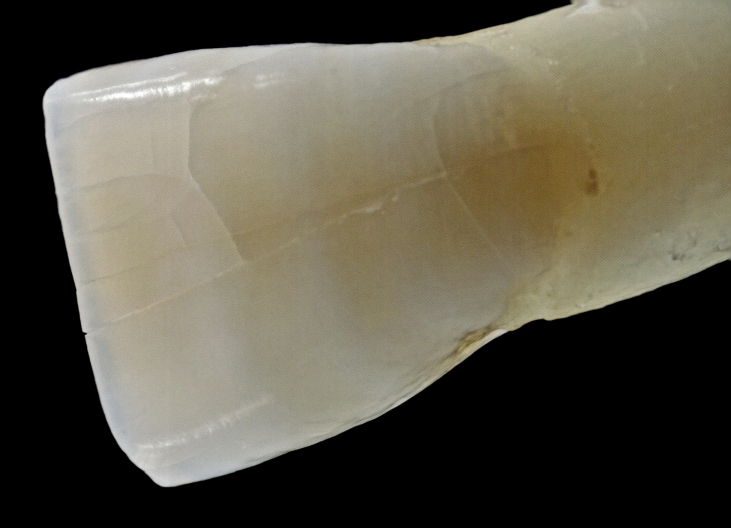

おそらくマメロンタイプから変化したテーパータイプの歯.

Taper type changed from Mamelon type (Probably).

Taper型天然牙也許是從Mamelon型變化而來.

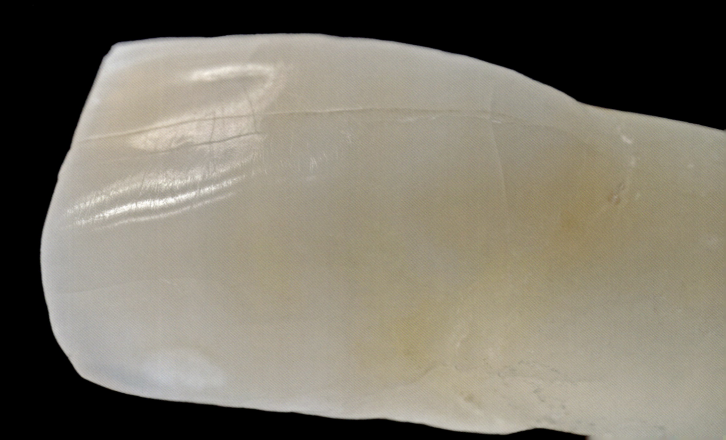

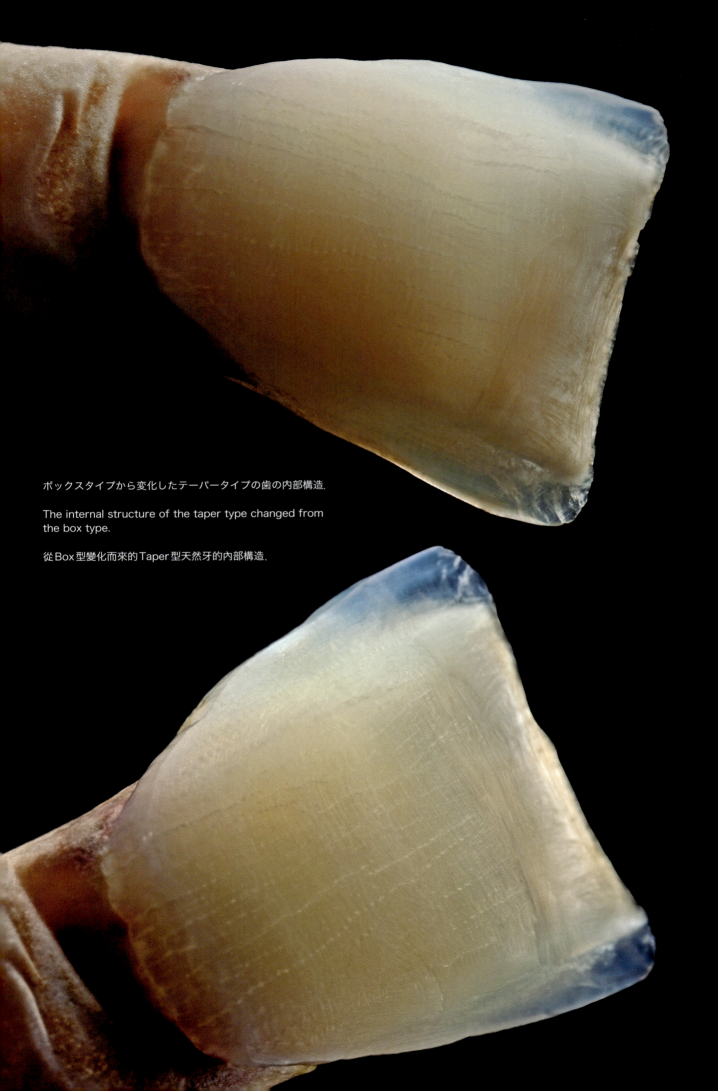

ボックスタイプから変化したテーパータイプの歯の内部構造.

The internal structure of the taper type changed from the box type.

從Box型變化而來的Taper型天然牙的內部構造.

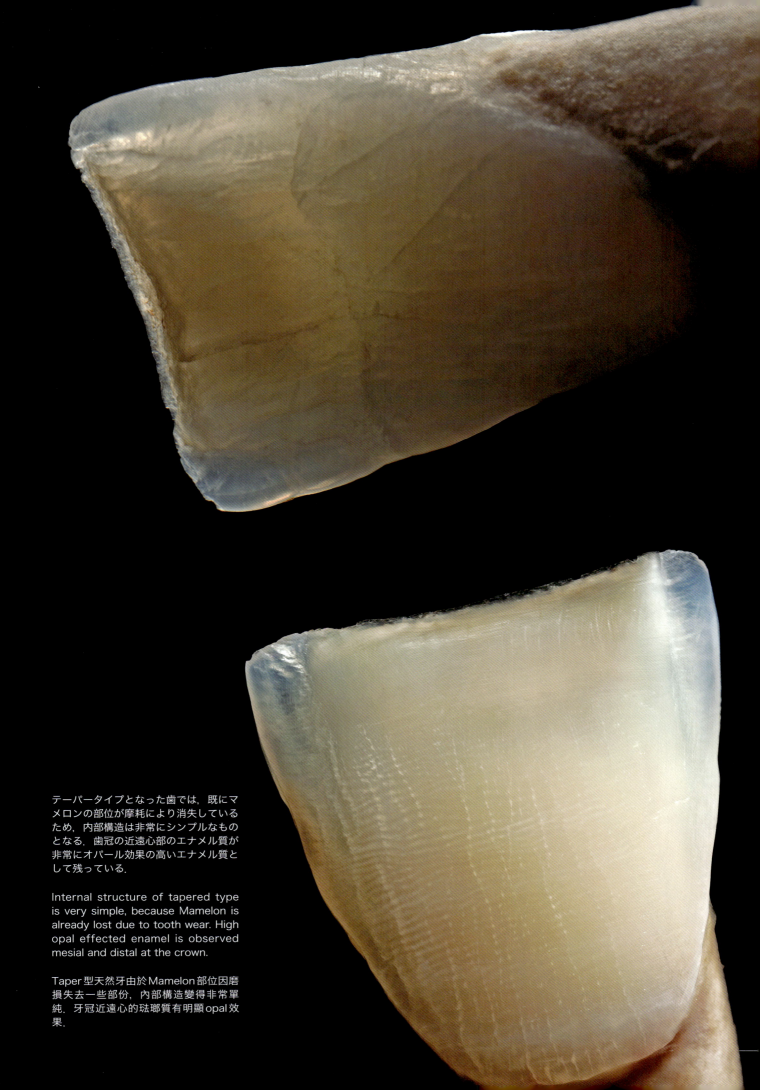

テーパータイプとなった歯では，既にマメロンの部位が摩耗により消失しているため，内部構造は非常にシンプルなものとなる．歯冠の近遠心部のエナメル質が非常にオパール効果の高いエナメル質として残っている．

Internal structure of tapered type is very simple, because Mamelon is already lost due to tooth wear. High opal effected enamel is observed mesial and distal at the crown.

Taper型天然牙由於Mamelon部位因磨損失去一些部份，內部構造變得非常單純．牙冠近遠心的琺瑯質有明顯opal效果．

Taper Type Linked to Palatal

テーパータイプの歯の唇側と舌側の連動性.

Relationship between labial and lingual side of the taper type.

Taper型天然牙唇側與舌側的相關性.

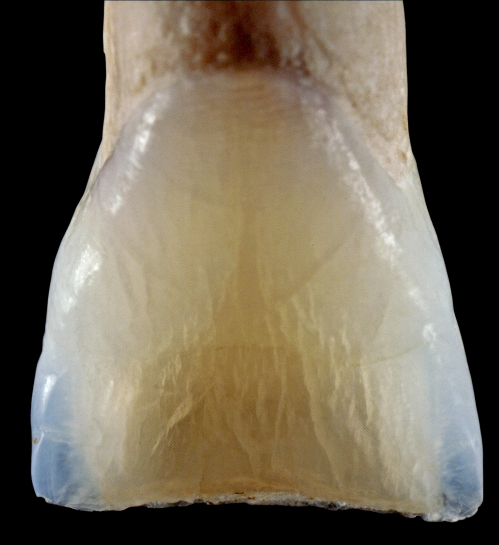

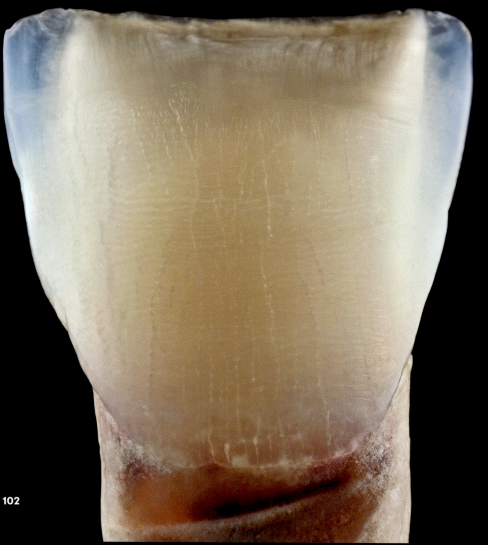

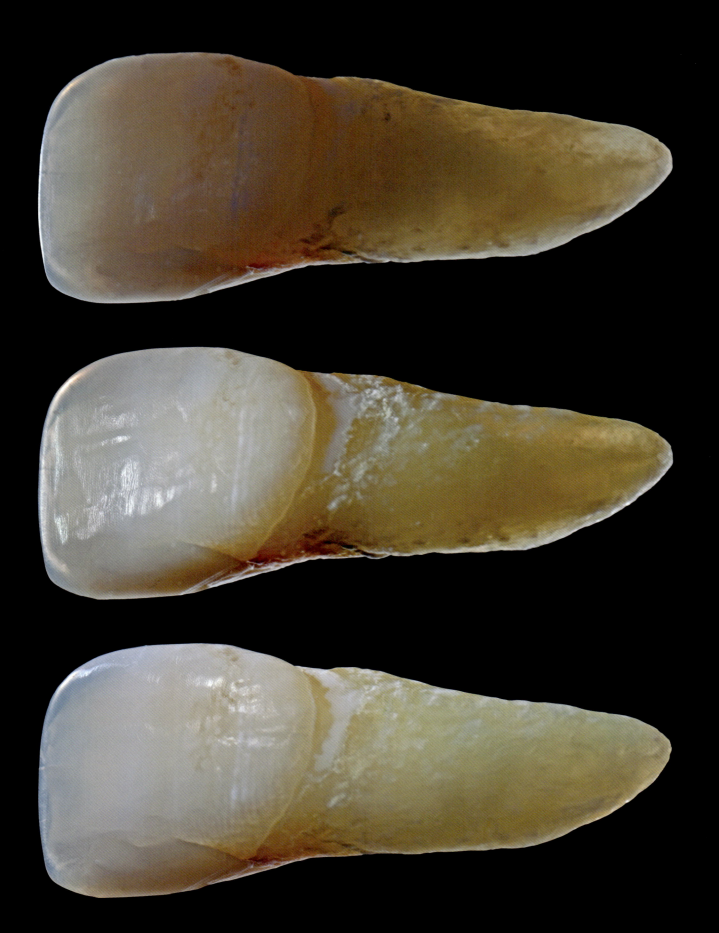

摩耗していないボックスタイプの歯の色調.

The tooth color of Box type without tooth wear.

沒有經過磨耗的Box型天然牙色調.

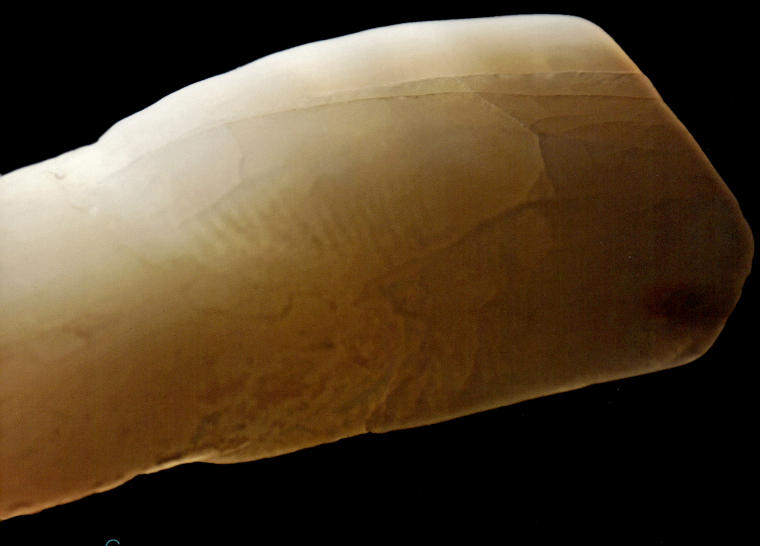

Part 6

Enamel

歯は月と同様，光がなければ輝くことはない．

The teeth are never shining without the light as the moon.

天然牙如同月娘，沒有了光就看不到她的皎然．

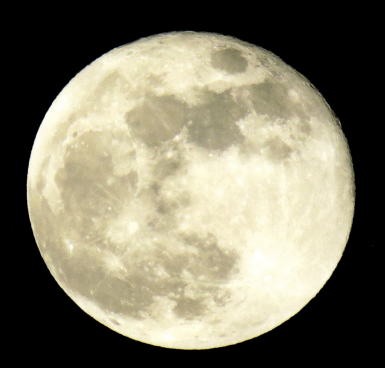

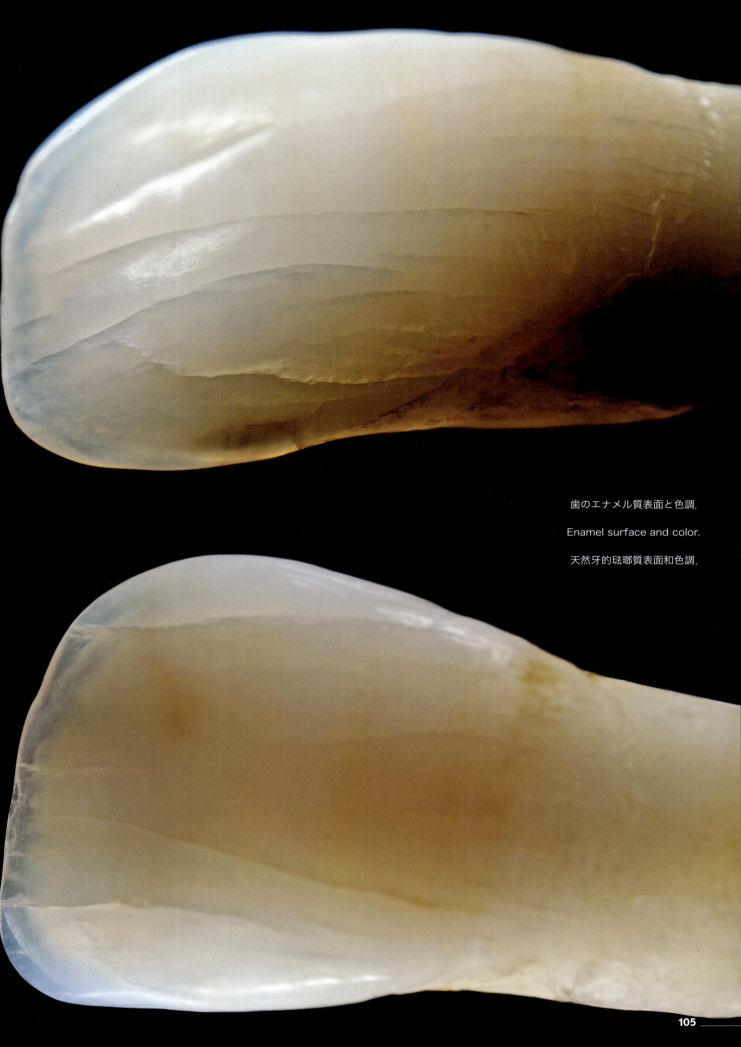

歯のエナメル質表面と色調.
Enamel surface and color.
天然牙的琺瑯質表面和色調.

歯は摩耗することにより切縁部のエナメル質の透明性にも変化が生じる.

The transparency of the incisal edge change by tooth wear.

因磨耗造成切緣的琺瑯質透明性產生變化.

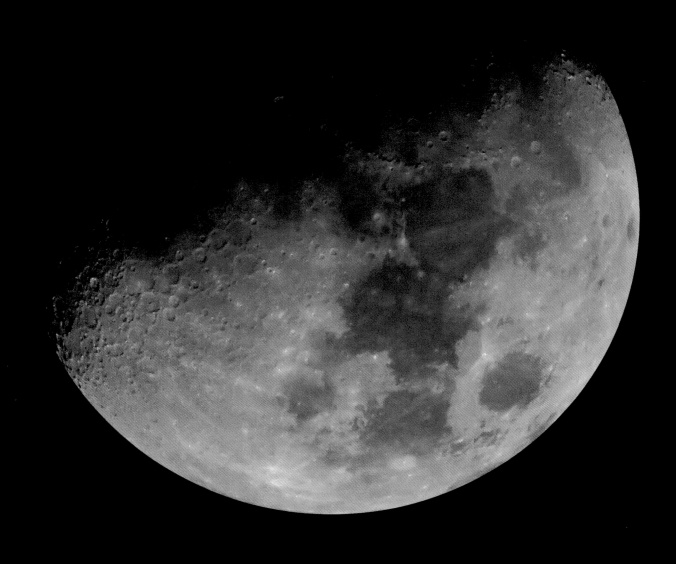

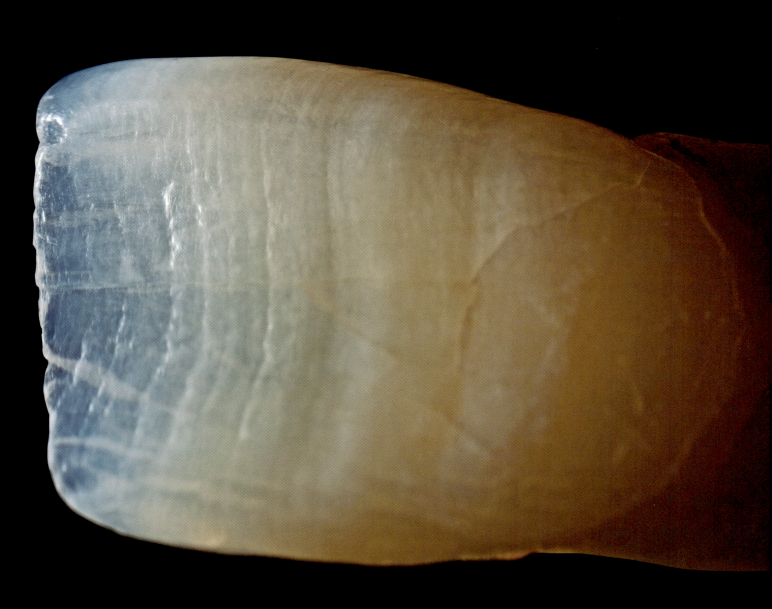

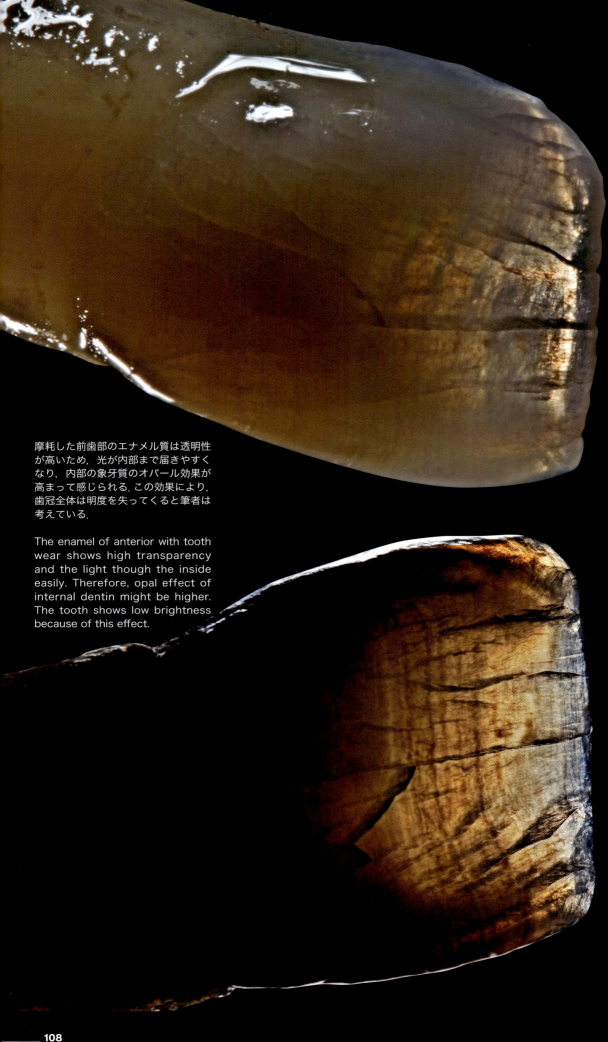

摩耗した前歯部のエナメル質は透明性が高いため，光が内部まで届きやすくなり，内部の象牙質のオパール効果が高まって感じられる．この効果により，歯冠全体は明度を失ってくると筆者は考えている．

The enamel of anterior with tooth wear shows high transparency and the light though the inside easily. Therefore, opal effect of internal dentin might be higher. The tooth shows low brightness because of this effect.

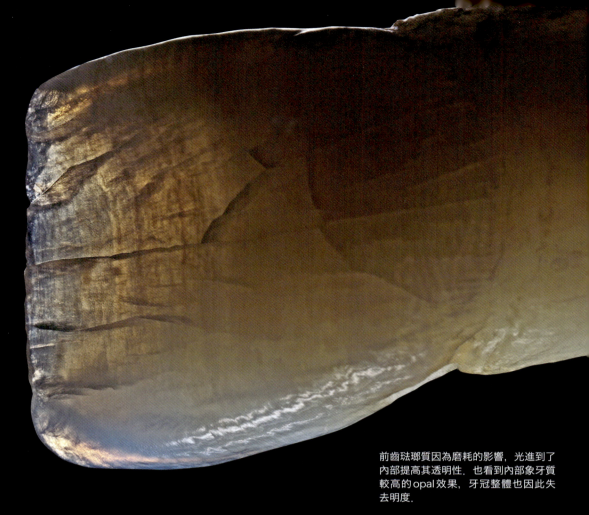

前齒琺瑯質因為磨耗的影響，光進到了內部提高其透明性，也看到內部象牙質較高的 opal 效果，牙冠整體也因此失去明度。

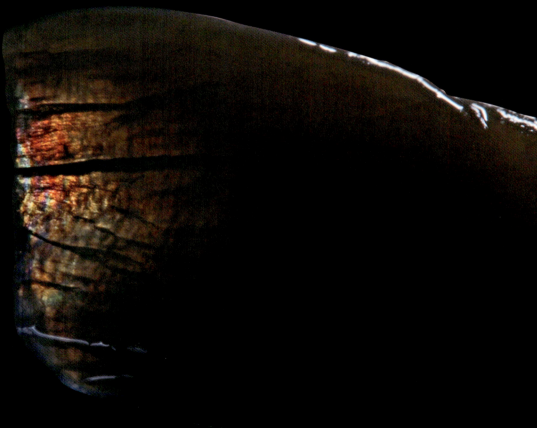

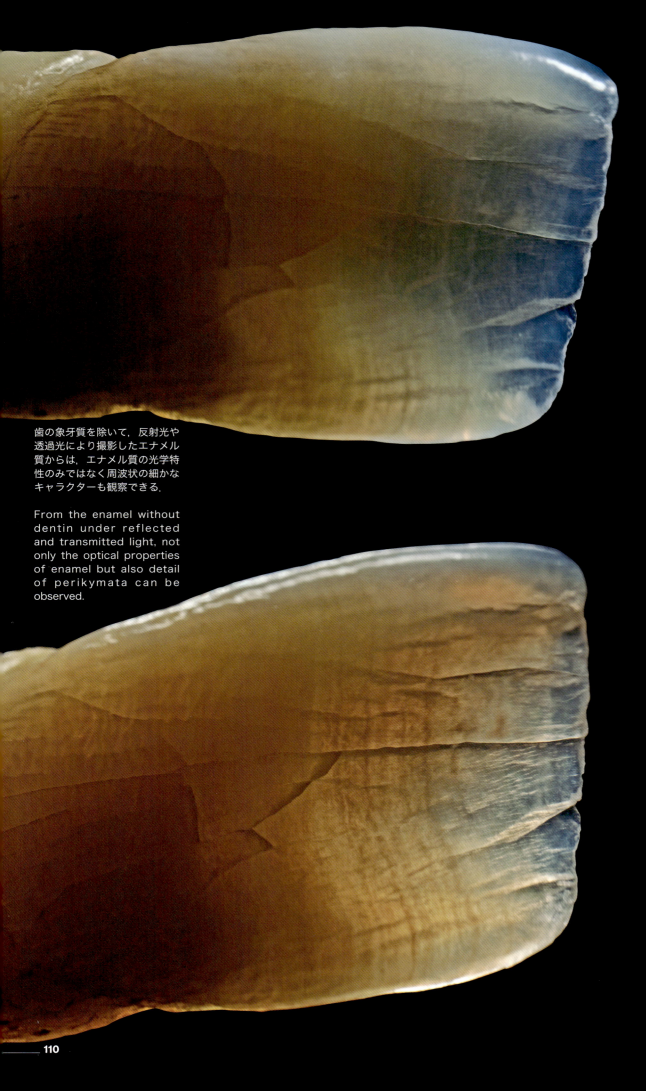

歯の象牙質を除いて，反射光や透過光により撮影したエナメル質からは，エナメル質の光学特性のみではなく周波状の細かなキャラクターも観察できる．

From the enamel without dentin under reflected and transmitted light, not only the optical properties of enamel but also detail of perikymata can be observed.

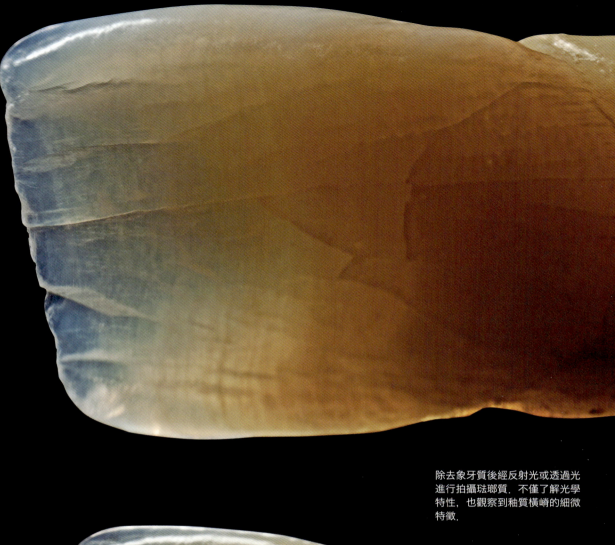

除去象牙質後經反射光或透過光進行拍攝琺瑯質．不僅了解光學特性，也觀察到釉質橫嵴的細微特徵．

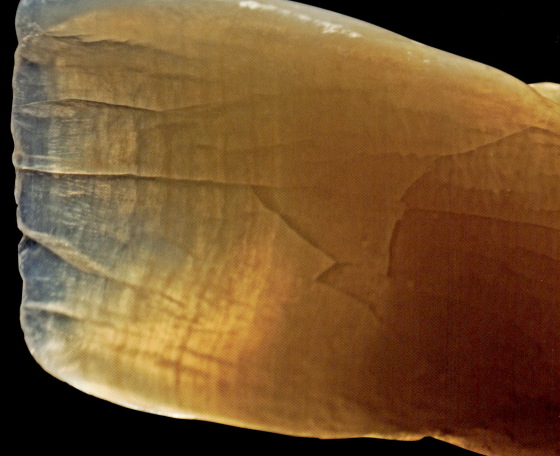

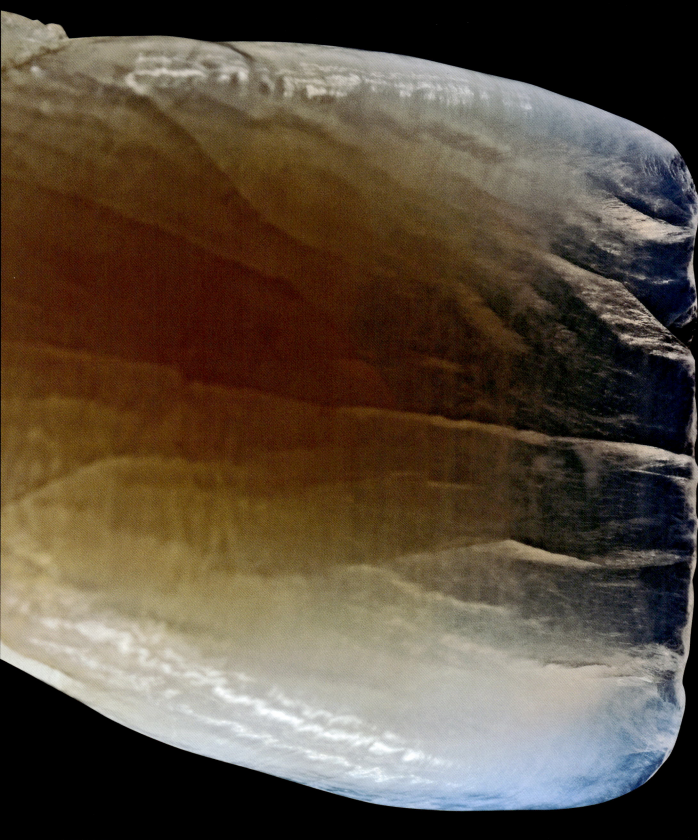

歯の象牙質を除いた状態で，エナメル質の側方からの反射光により撮影したエナメル質．

Observation from the surface of enamel without dentin under reflected light.

除去象牙質後，從側面照射反射光所進行的琺瑯質拍攝

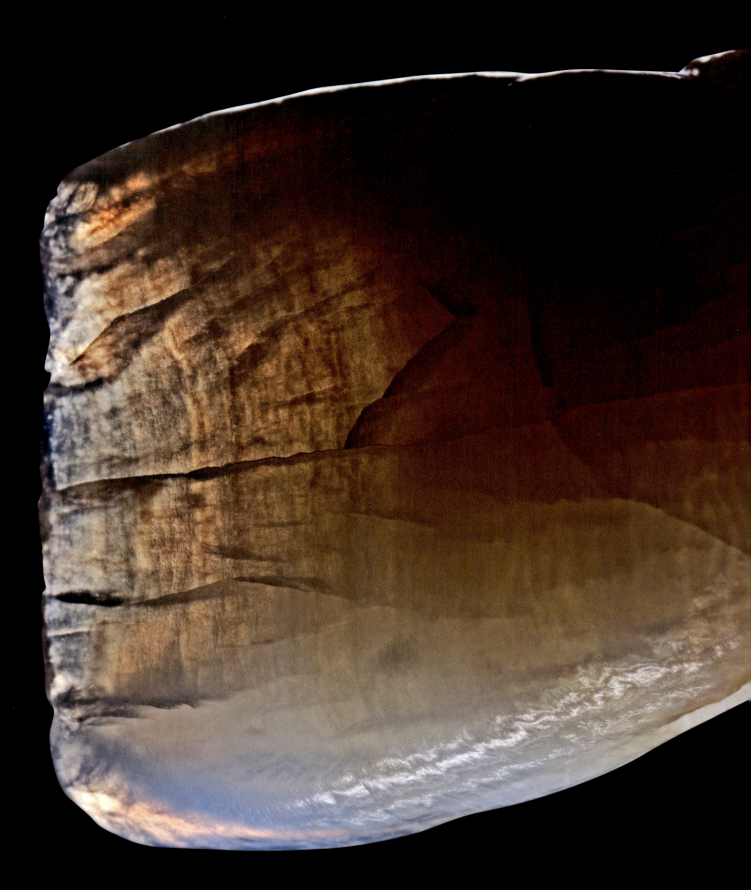

歯の象牙質を除いた状態で，完全な透過光により撮影したエナメル質．

Observation from the surface of enamel without dentin under transmitted light.

除去象牙質後，以透過光進行琺瑯質拍攝．

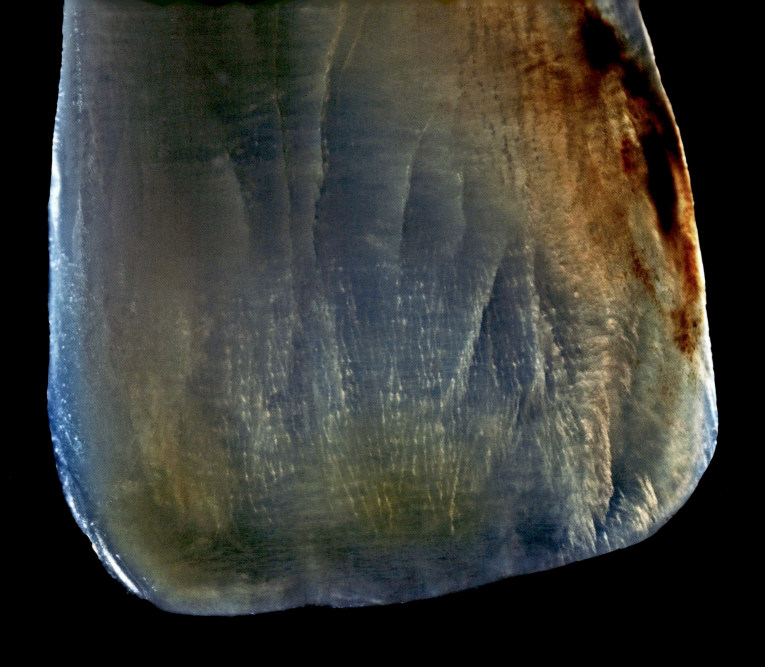

歯の象牙質を除いた状態で，エナメル質の左右側方からの反射光により撮影したエナメル質．

Observation from the surface of enamel without dentin under reflected light from reft and right side.

除去象牙質後，從左右兩側的反射光進行琺瑯質拍攝．

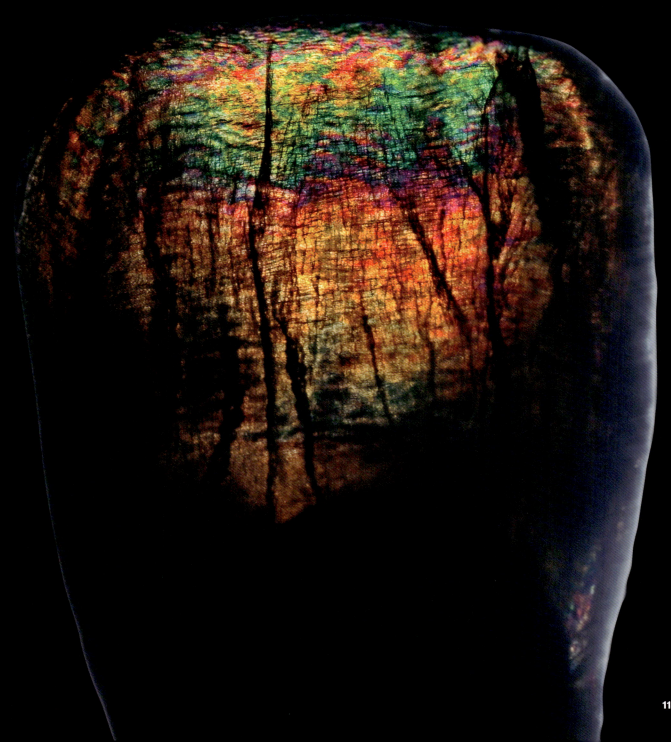

歯のエナメル質には，光学特性による色調効果と微細な表面性状による色彩効果がある．

The enamel shows a color effect affected by optical and morphological properties.

琺瑯質光學特性產生的色調效果，以及細微表面性狀產生的色彩．

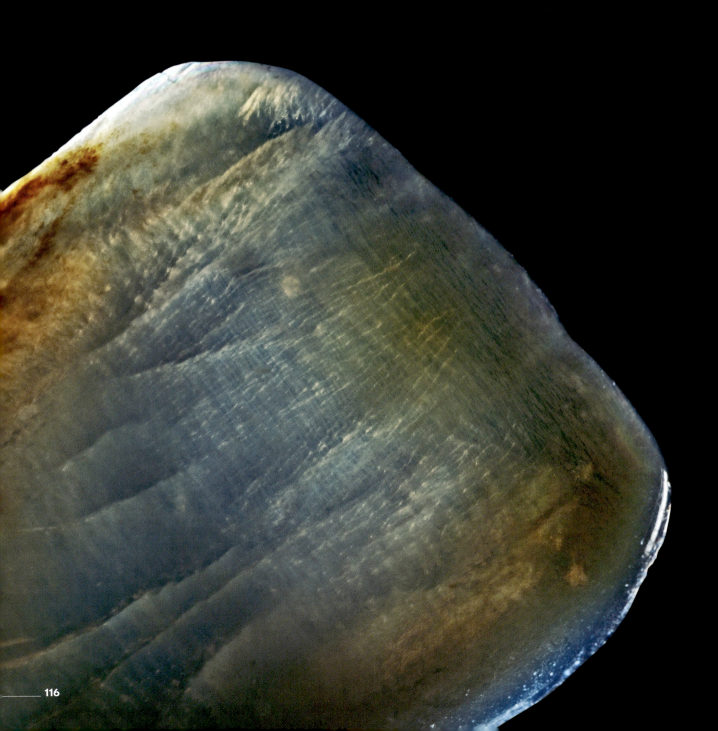

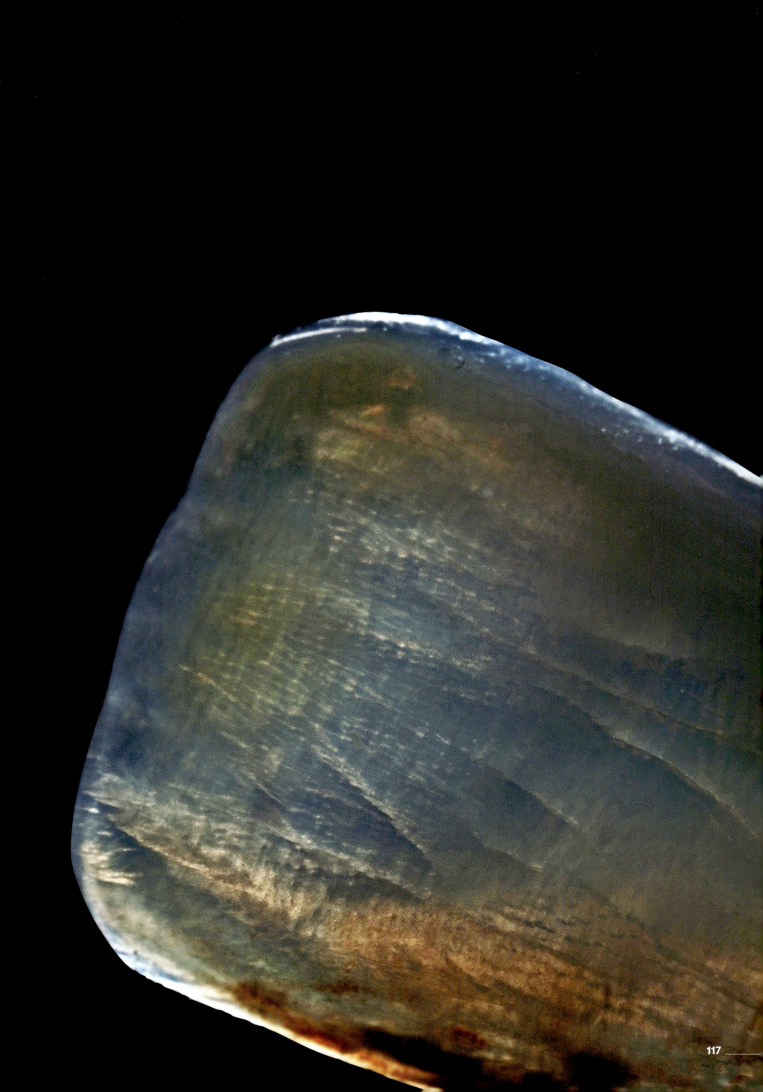

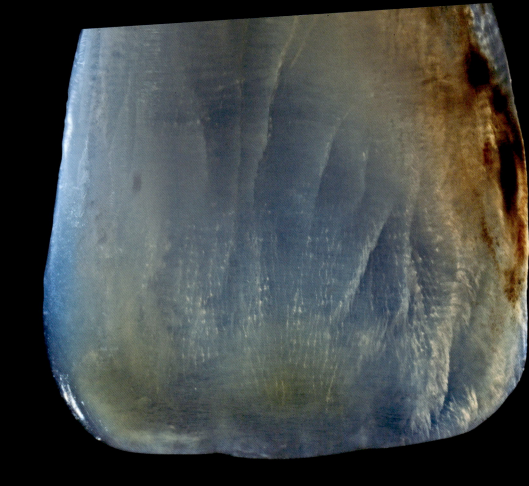

歯のエナメル質の虹色の効果.

Iridescent effect of enamel.

琺瑯質的虹彩效果.

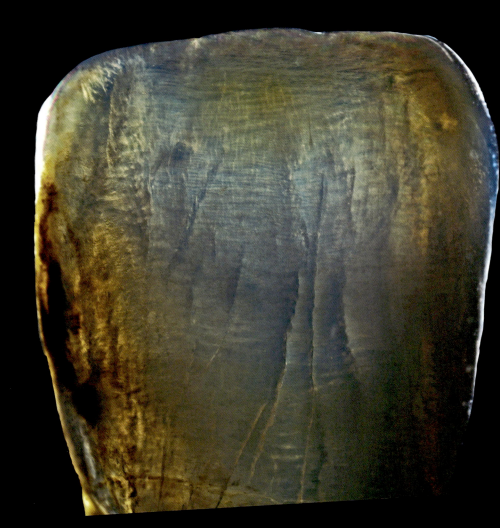

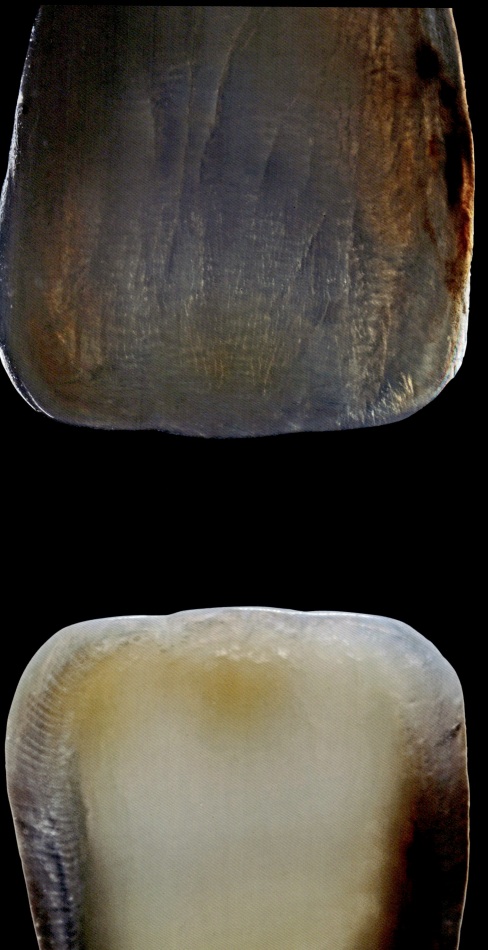

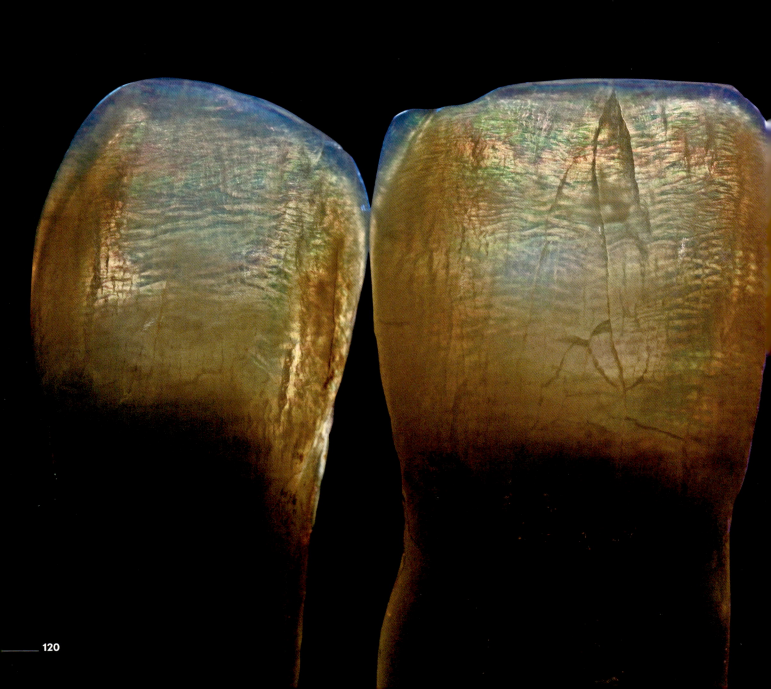

歯の象牙質を削除したエナメル質の虹色の効果.
Iridescent effect of enamel without dentin.
除去象牙質後的琺瑯質虹彩效果

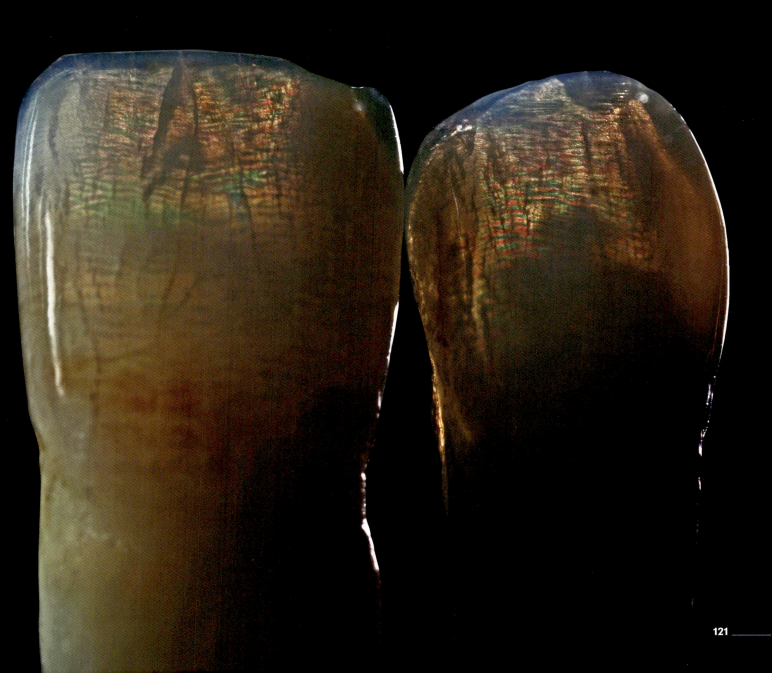

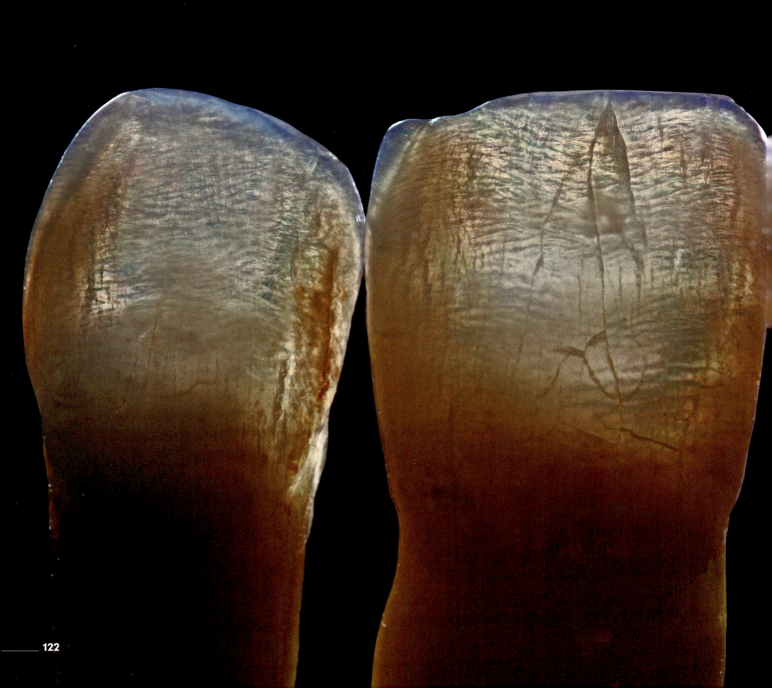

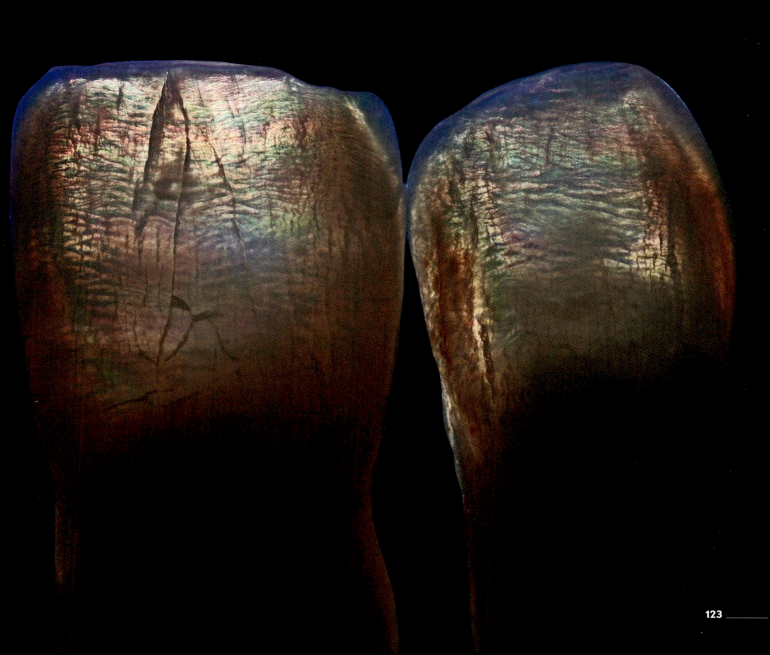

Part 7
Lateral incisor

上顎側切歯とその内部構造.

Internal and surface structure of maxillary lateral incisor.

上顎側門齒及其內部構造.

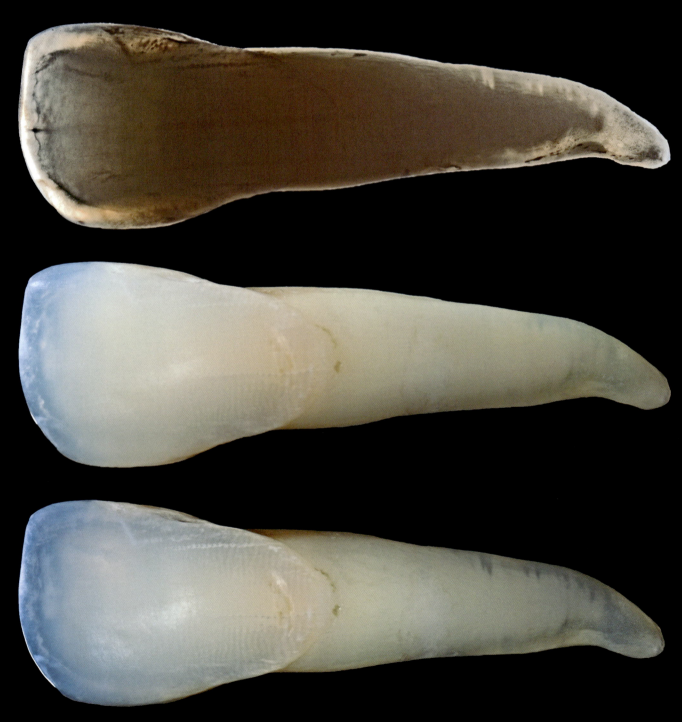

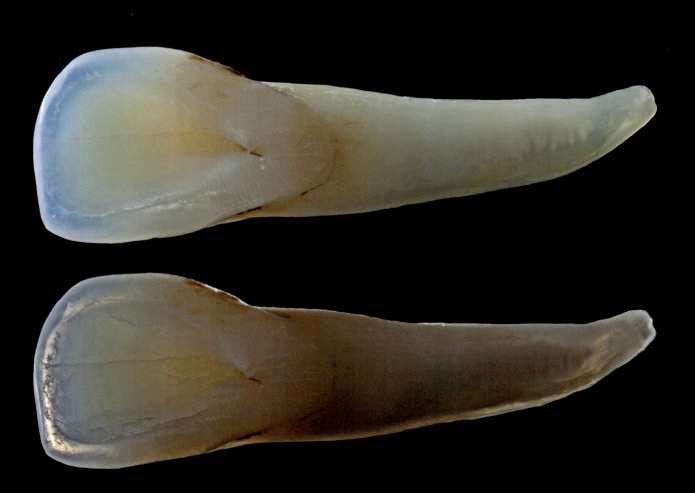

マメロンタイプの上顎側切歯の内部構造.

Internal structure of the Mamelon type of maxillary lateral incisor.

Mamelon型上顎側門齒的內部構造.

ボックスタイプの上顎側切歯の内部構造.

Internal structure of the Box type of maxillary lateral incisor.

Box型上顎側門齒的內部構造.

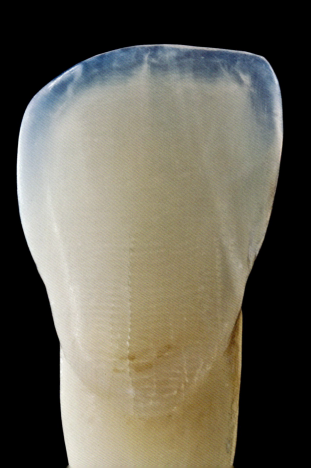
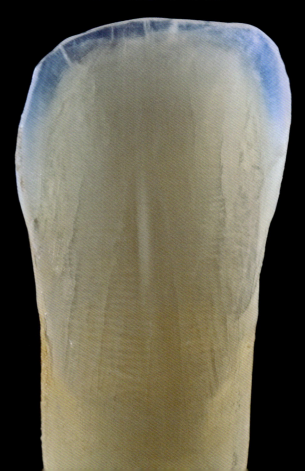

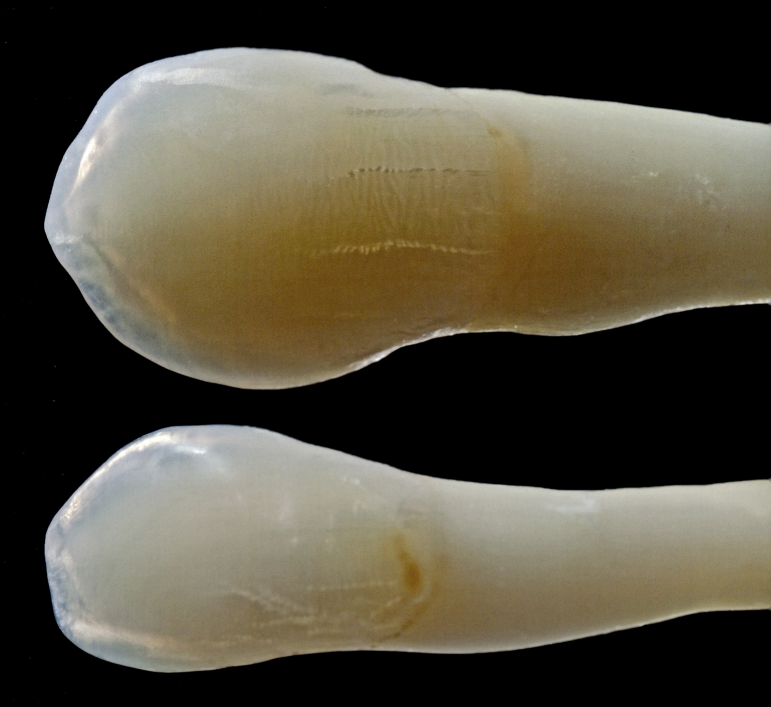

Part 8
Canine

上顎犬歯と下顎犬歯の唇側と舌側.

Labial and lingual side of the maxillary canine and mandibular canine.

上下顎犬齒的唇側和舌側.

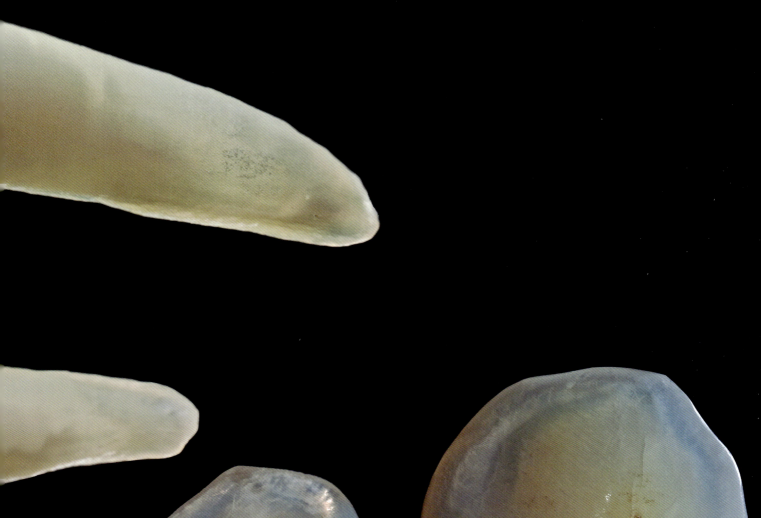

上顎犬歯の唇側のエナメル質を削除した内部構造と舌側色調.

Internal structure and lingual color of maxillary canine eliminated from labial enamel.

上顎犬齒唇側除去琺瑯質後的內部構造和舌側色調.

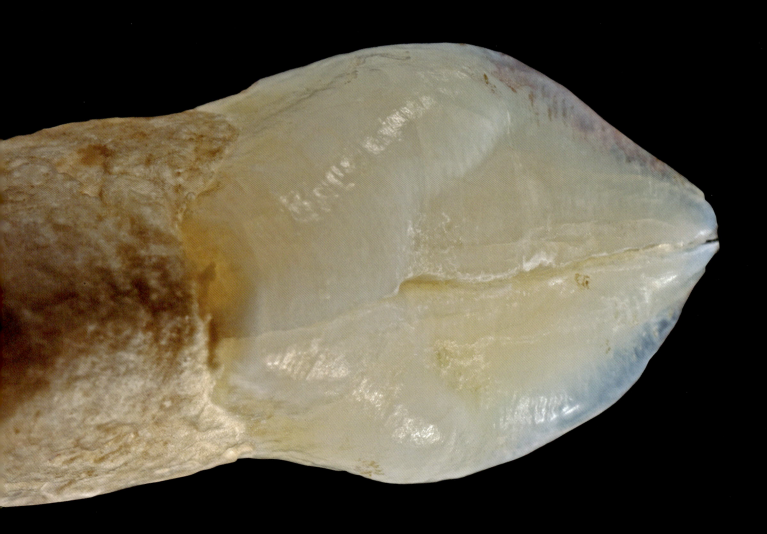

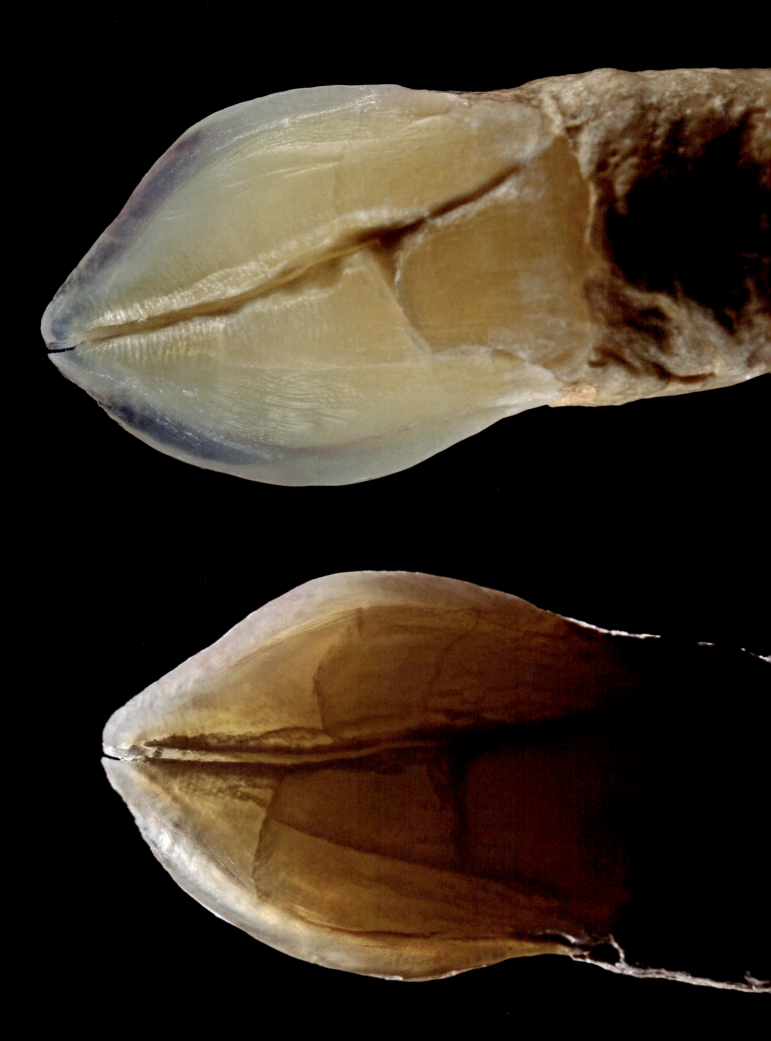

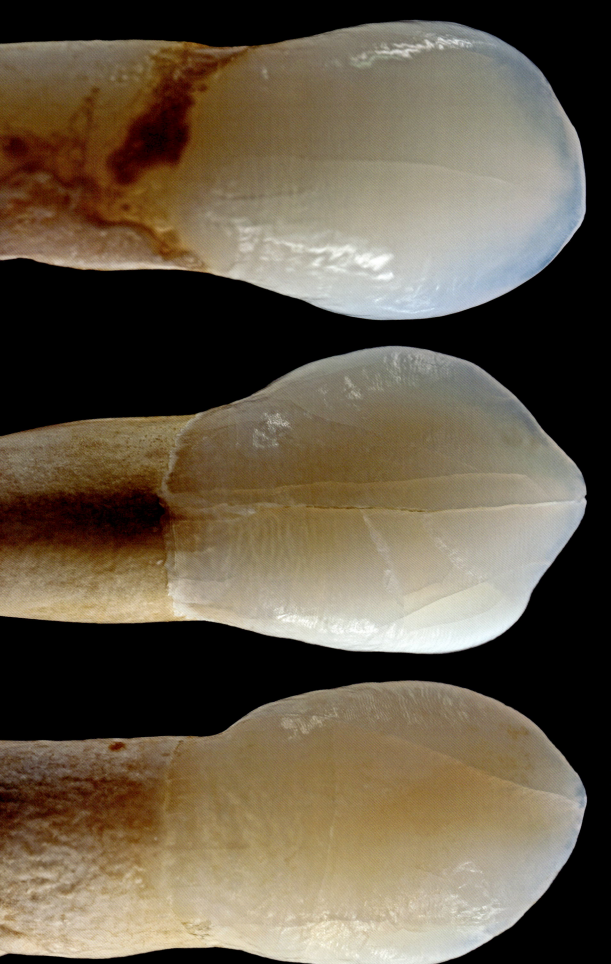

上顎犬歯のタイプ別の特徴
→テーパータイプ
→尖形タイプ
→米粒型タイプ

Characteristic on different type of maxillary canine.
→Taper type.
→Sharp type.
→Oval (rice shape) type.

上顎犬歯特徴分類
→Taper型
→尖型
→米粒型

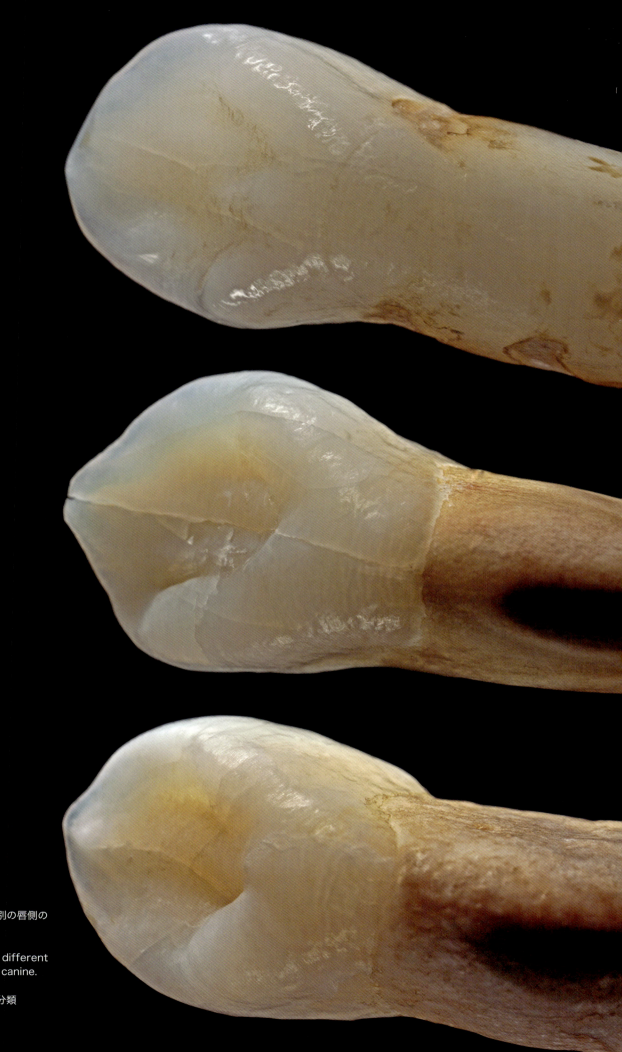

上顎犬歯のタイプ別の唇側の形状.

Labial shape on different type of maxillary canine.

上顎犬歯唇側型態分類

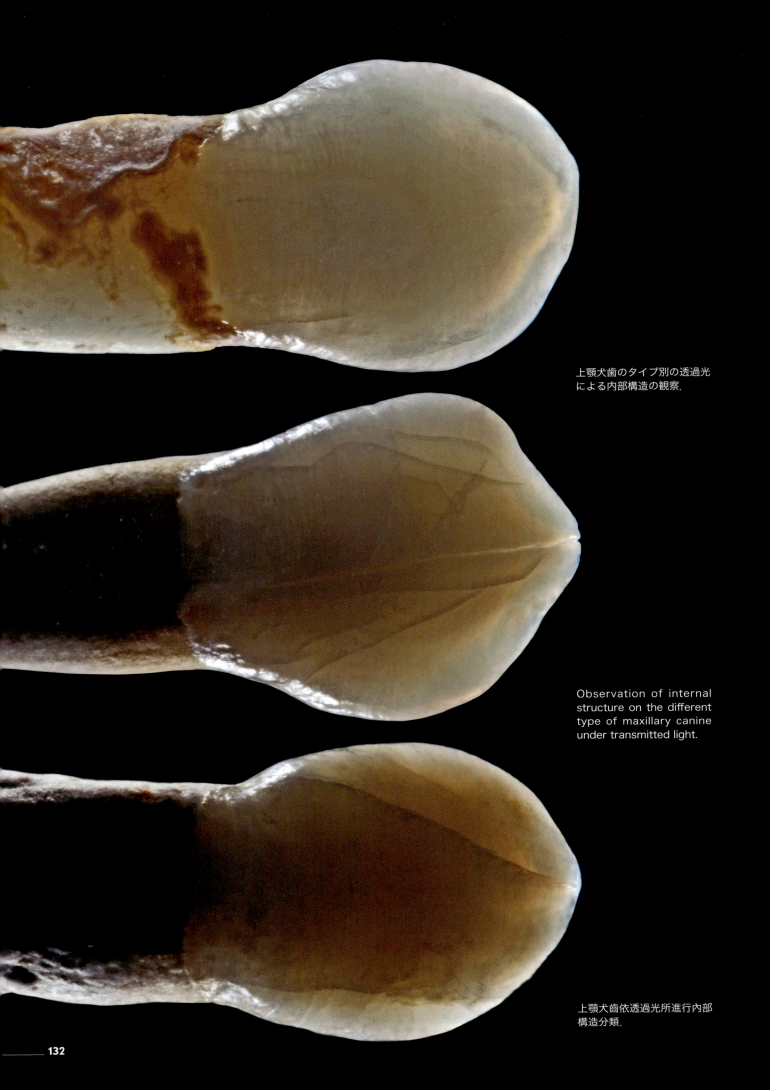

上顎犬歯のタイプ別の透過光による内部構造の観察.

Observation of internal structure on the different type of maxillary canine under transmitted light.

上顎犬歯依透過光所進行內部構造分類.

上顎犬歯のタイプ別の左右からの透過光による内部構造の観察.

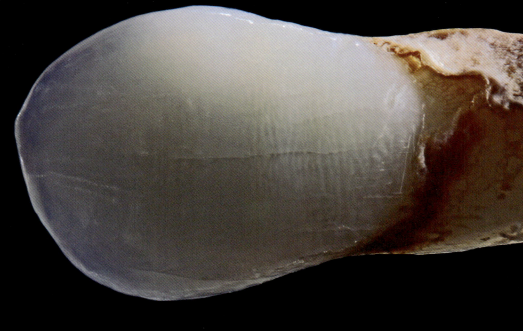

Observation from the internal structure on different type of maxillary canine under reflected light from reft and right side.

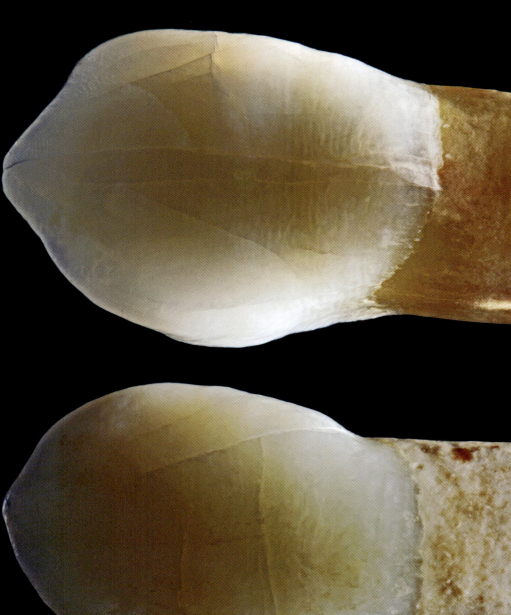

上顎犬歯左右透過光所進行內部構造分類.

Lower anteriores

下顎中切歯は若年層もしくは切縁での咬合がなされていない場合を除いて，切縁が直線的に摩耗していることが多い．また，左右の隣接面のエナメル質は歯のコンタクトポイントより下まで（おおよそ歯冠の2/3まで）観察できる．

Many lower anterior teeth show straight wear at the incisal edge, except younger age and/or open bite. In addition, the left and right of the enamel can be observed under the contact point (Roughly it can be observed up to two-thirds of the crown).

下顎中門齒多是有呈現直線的磨耗，除了較年輕的族群或是切緣尚未咬合的族群以外．另外可觀察到左右鄰接面的琺瑯質是在contact point下方（約在牙冠2/3）．

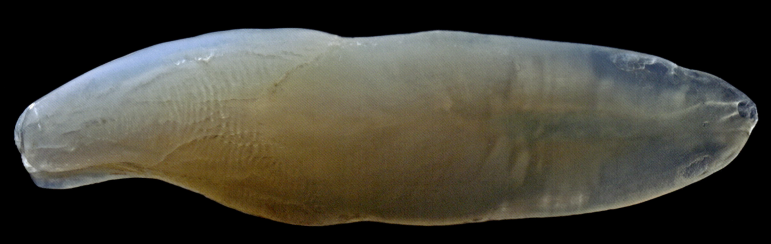

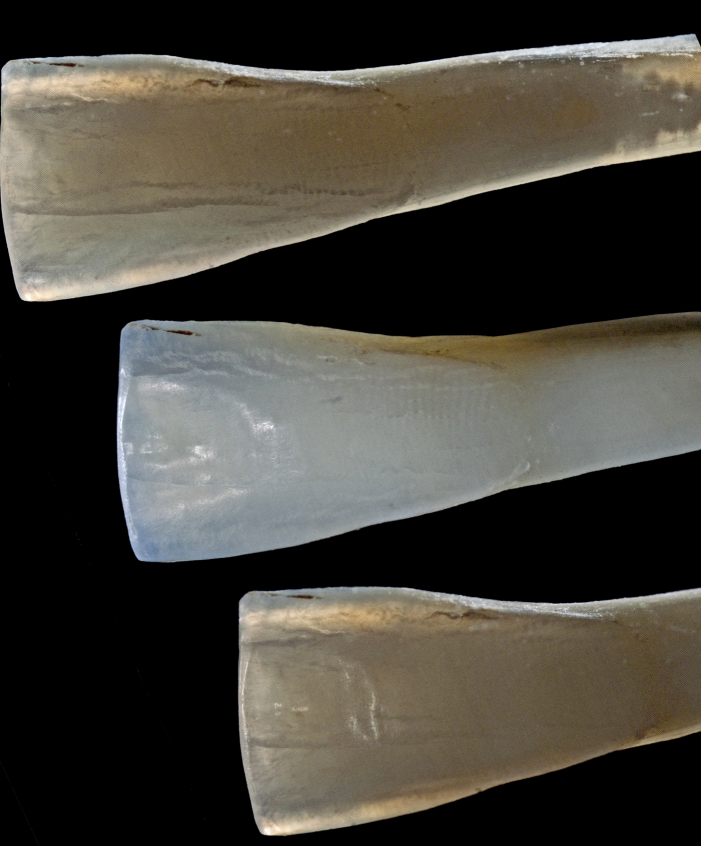

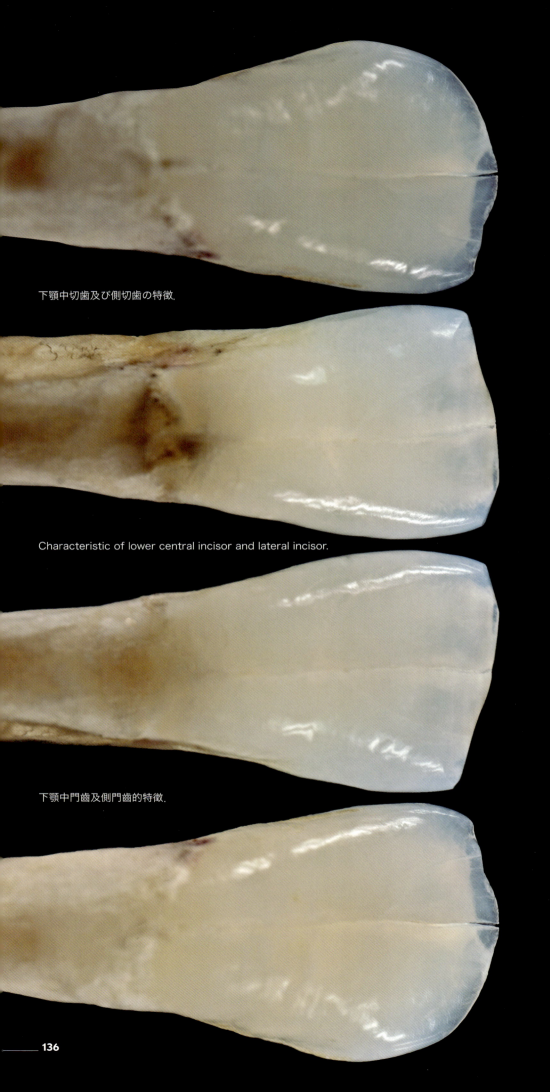

下顎中切歯及び側切歯の特徴.

Characteristic of lower central incisor and lateral incisor.

下顎中門齒及側門齒的特徵.

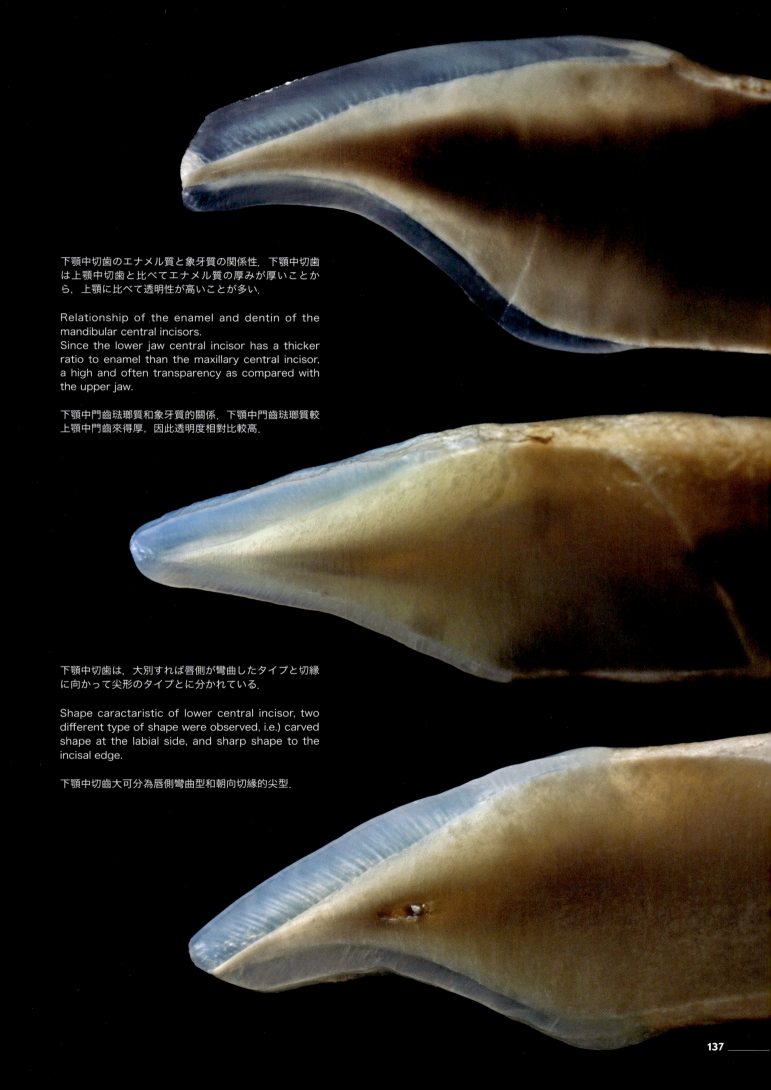

下顎中切歯のエナメル質と象牙質の関係性．下顎中切歯は上顎中切歯と比べてエナメル質の厚みが厚いことから，上顎に比べて透明性が高いことが多い．

Relationship of the enamel and dentin of the mandibular central incisors.
Since the lower jaw central incisor has a thicker ratio to enamel than the maxillary central incisor, a high and often transparency as compared with the upper jaw.

下顎中門齒琺瑯質和象牙質的關係．下顎中門齒琺瑯質較上顎中門齒來得厚，因此透明度相對比較高．

下顎中切歯は，大別すれば唇側が彎曲したタイプと切縁に向かって尖形のタイプとに分かれている．

Shape caractaristic of lower central incisor, two different type of shape were observed, i.e.) carved shape at the labial side, and sharp shape to the incisal edge.

下顎中切齒大可分為唇側彎曲型和朝向切緣的尖型．

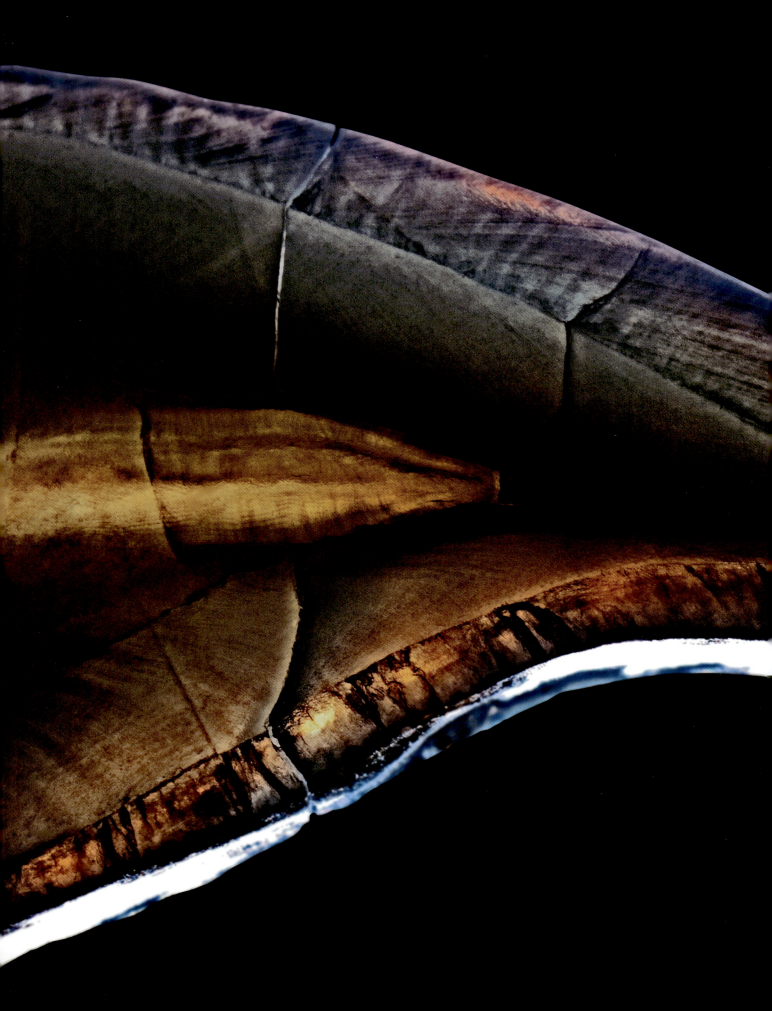

Appendix

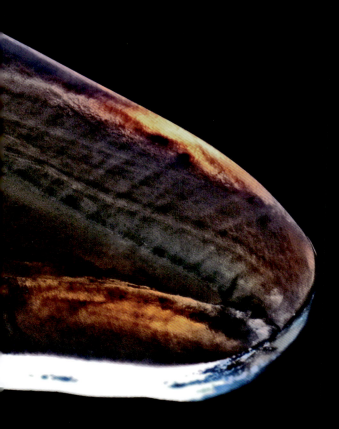

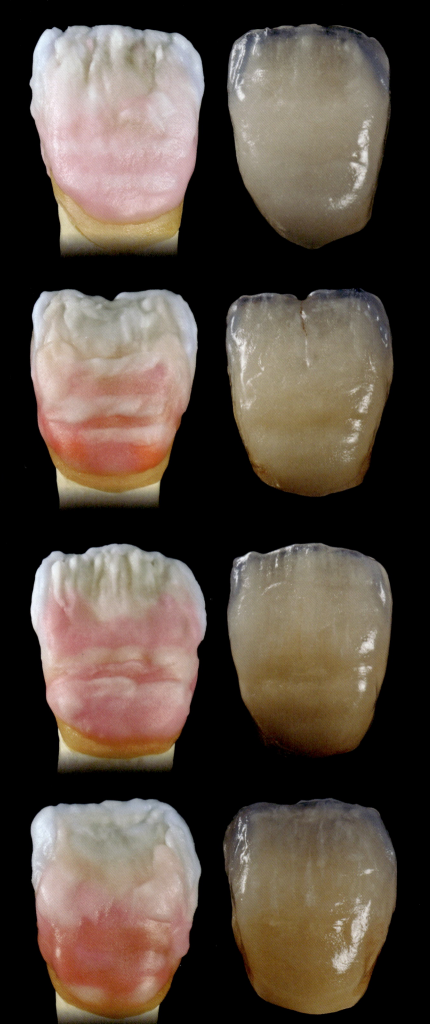

Mamelon type Layering

Mamelon Devil type Layering

Box type Layering

Box Devil type Layering

Appendix

Harmony with Soft Tissue

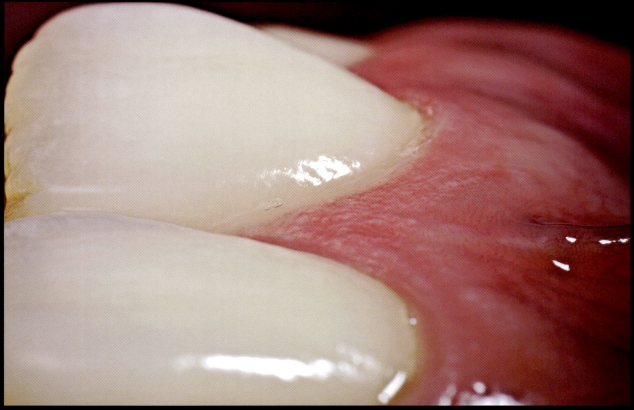

▲我々歯科技工士は，臨在歯の色調にマッチし，歯周組織と調和するような形態が整った補綴物の製作を模索する．そして，歯周組織が補綴物を天然歯であると"勘違い"してくれることを望んでいる．

Texture

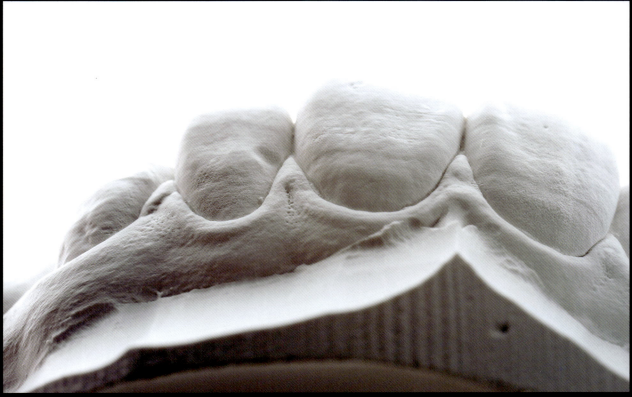

▲もちろん，色調は審美補綴において重要なテーマであるが，歯の形態及び表面性情の観察・表現もまた色調再現にとって必要な要件である．

Special Thanks

英文翻訳

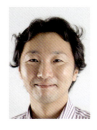

Dr. 新谷明一　Akikazu Shinya, DDS, PhD

日本歯科大学生命歯学部歯科補綴学第2講座 准教授
フィンランド・トゥルク大学補綴・生体材料学講座 研究員
香港大学牙医学院牙科物質学 客員准教授

1999年 日本歯科大学歯学部 卒業
2003年 日本歯科大学大学院歯学研究科臨床系 修了
2006年 日本歯科大学生命歯学部歯科補綴学第2講座 助手
2008年 フィンランド・トゥルク大学補綴・生体材料学講座大学院 入学
2009年 香港大学牙医学院牙科物質学 客員 准教授
2010年 日本歯科大学生命歯学部歯科補綴学第2講座 講師
2015年 日本歯科大学生命歯学部歯科補綴学第2講座 准教授
2016年 日本歯科大学生命歯学部歯科補綴学第2講座 副部長

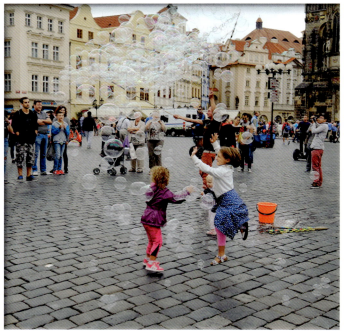

プラハ，旧市街広場にて　　　Photo by Akikazu Shinya

繁体中文翻訳

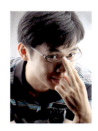

RDT. 李 唯嘉（Sam Li）

2011年 日本の歯科技工士免許 取得
2013年 Daladontics Orthodontics Lab 勤務
2014年 台湾の歯科技工士免許 取得
2014年 株式会社 AYM

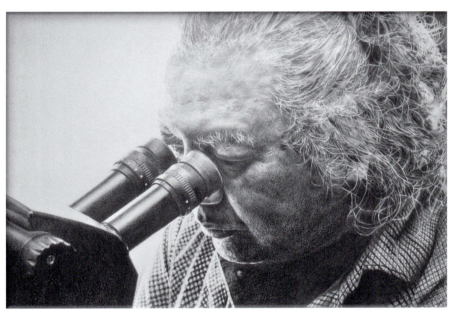

山本尚吾牙技師　　　　　　　　　　　Pencil Drawing by Sam Li

- -

and Author…

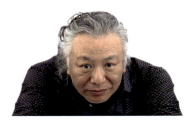

Show Yamamoto

【著者略歴】
山本 尚吾（やま もと しょう ご）

1980年	愛媛県歯科技工学校卒業
2007年	art&experience BeR（ビー エ アール）開設
2001年	VOCE Ceramist Club 主宰
2006年	VOCE C.C Claymore 主宰
	Claude Sieber 氏主宰，art & experience メンバー
	CAMLOG インプラント 認定講師
	CAMLOG インターナショナルコングレス（カナダ・モントレー）登壇
2007年	VITA 社 masterlab 認定
2008年	BEGO Crown Bridge Ambassdor
2009年	日本歯科審美学会 認定講師
2010年	Sirona CEREC in Lab Evangelist
2015年	IADDM Active Member
	Massironi Study Club スピーカー
	AMED スピーカー
	CEREC Asia トレーナー
	Leica experience Lab 認定

その他，日本国際歯科大会シンポジウムに多数回登壇．国内外の学術誌・商業誌に約200本の論文を執筆．「セラミックスの色調とフレーム材の強度及び色調への影響について」「口腔内の歯列におけるポジションと歯冠形態について」を主要なテーマとする．

Impact Color and internal shape of Anteriores

ISBN978-4-263-46213-3

2017年4月10日　第1版第1刷発行

著　者　山　本　尚　吾
発行者　白　石　泰　夫

発行所　医歯薬出版株式会社

〒113-8612　東京都文京区本駒込 1-7-10
TEL.（03）5395-7635（編集）・7630（販売）
FAX.（03）5395-7639（編集）・7633（販売）
http://www.ishiyaku.co.jp/
郵便振替番号　00190-5-13816

乱丁・落丁の際はお取り替えいたします　　印刷・第一印刷所／製本・榎本製本
Ⓒ Ishiyaku Publishers, Inc., 2017. Printed in Japan

本書の複製権・翻訳権・翻案権・上映権・譲渡権・貸与権・公衆送信権（送信可能化権を含む）・口述権は，医歯薬出版㈱が保有します．
本書を無断で複製する行為（コピー，スキャン，デジタルデータ化など）は，「私的使用のための複製」などの著作権法上の限られた例外を除き禁じられています．また私的使用に該当する場合であっても，請負業者等の第三者に依頼し上記の行為を行うことは違法となります．

JCOPY ＜(社)出版者著作権管理機構　委託出版物＞
本書をコピーやスキャン等により複写される場合は，そのつど事前に(社)出版者著作権管理機構（電話 03-3513-6969，FAX 03-3513-6979，e-mail: info@jcopy.or.jp）の許諾を得てください．